The GIANT in Me

A Memoir

BY:
DANIEL HAWTHORNE
With Patricia Garber

Copyright 2021 by Patricia Garber LLC

All rights reserved. No part of this book may be reproduced or transmitted in any form or by any means, electronic or mechanical, including photocopying, recording, or by any information storage and retrieval system, without permission in writing from the copyright owner.

ISBN-13: 979-8-9862198-0-6
LCCN: 2022909106
Jungle Room Press
Patricia Garber LLC
eternflame@yahoo.com

Events in this book are shared to the best of the author's knowledge. To protect the privacy of others, names and details may have been changed. And while all events are true, in some cases, the timeline has been shifted for the sake of the story flow.

Disclaimer
Daniel W. Hawthorne and Patricia L. Garber are not doctors, or medical professionals. The views expressed are those of the author's alone and should not be taken as expert instruction or commands. All readers are responsible for his or her own actions.

Adherence to all applicable laws and regulations, including international, federal, state, and local governing professional licensing, business practices, advertising, and all other aspects of doing business in the US, Canada, or any other jurisdiction is the sole responsibility of the purchaser or reader.

Neither the author nor the publisher assumes any responsibility or liability whatsoever on the behalf of the purchaser or reader of these materials.

Any perceived slight of any individual or organization is purely unintentional.

Book design by Alexander Von Ness at Nessgraphica
Editing and formatting by Ceri Savage at Savage Edits
Back photo by Jeremy Drury, New York City

This book was printed in the United State of America.

DEDICATION

Patricia; will you marry me, my angel, my soul mate?

Contents

Author's Note 7

Introduction 11

    Chapter One. Food: The happy times 17

    Chapter Two. Growing pains 25

    Chapter Three. Love and Radio 37

    Chapter Four. Home at the bottom 51

    Chapter Five. Get real 63

    Chapter Six. Find Support 73

    Chapter Seven. Baby steps 91

    Chapter Eight. The plan 105

    Chapter Nine. Expect bumps 117

    Chapter Ten. Find your inner strength 127

    Chapter Eleven. Love yourself 139

    Chapter Twelve. Get Cooking 151

    Chapter Thirteen. Give back 167

    Chapter Fourteen. A journey in words 181

    Chapter Fifteen. Dreaming 191

    Chapter Sixteen. Consequences 203

    Chapter Seventeen. Confidence 217

Chapter Eighteen. The Move 227

Chapter Nineteen. Second chances 245

Chapter Twenty. Conclusions 257

Addendum 265

Acknowledgments 275

From Patricia Garber 281

Other Books by Patricia Garber 285

In Loving Memory 287

Author's Note

THREE YEARS, FOUR MONTHS, AND three days; that is how long I lived as a morbidly obese man. That's 1,220 humiliating days, 1,7567,482 minutes of hating myself to the point of wishing I'd simply disappear.

Then in October of 2013, a doctor said, "I cannot find a thing wrong with your blood work," and I watched as he hurriedly flipped through the pages on a clipboard. My breath held, waiting for him to find something, anything that would take away the happiness that filled my chest.

Twelve months prior, in 2012, I had been given a pending death sentence, when that same doctor predicted, "If you do not change your ways, you may not see fifty."

I was 48.

Two years to go, fatty, Beelzebub, my internal voice of doom, chirped in my ear.

It is grossly poetic and slightly ridiculous that I should name my inner conscience as a Philistine god, better known as a devil, but the title suited him.

Beelzebub was the voice I heard on that day in 2012, laughing, while the doctor announced my death as matter-of-factly as one calls kids to the supper table. Death by diabetes—a gourmet dish I'd rather not sample. And at that moment, nobody would have guessed

AUTHOR'S NOTE

that in just 360 days, I would step on a scale and chart a loss of well over 300 pounds. Nor that my blood work would show no further signs of death!

Dan Hawthorne was alive, and Beelzebub was dead.

Inside these pages you hold in your hand lies the key to how I got my life back, how I silenced my Beelzebub, and how you can silence that voice telling you it is too hard, you are not worth it, and nobody cares. And the worse joust yet? You are not loved.

Obese men and women live with these lies in a world trying to convince us we do not fit in; we do not look like everyone else. And we feel judged and alone.

I'm not a doctor; I have no certificates on my wall. I'm just a man who has lived most of his life obese in America. But I'm the one who understands the pain, the struggle, and I want to help you find peace again, love yourself again, and live a healthy and happy life. To shed the weight and sadness caused by obesity, we must first address why we are obese.

I know this may sound like some new-age gimmick, but I am not here to be your life savior, nor am I here to sell you a magic pill. I'm simply a food addict who's found a way to break the chains. How can I not share my journey? What kind of a man would I be if I did not try to help those struggling with many of the same demons I battle to this day?

And as I write these words in the summer of 2021, post-publication, I continue to use the methods mapped out inside these pages.

I will not lie to you, once a food addict, always a food addict. You won't read this book and suddenly be cured, and I encourage all to seek professional help when needed. What I am going to share with you is how I managed to keep my Beelzebub caged. How I learned to love myself and live a life of purpose again. And if one tool inside these pages helps you, I have done my job.

We will laugh together. We may cry a little too. And in the end, I pray that you not just desire a healthier life, but you believe it's within your reach. I want you to crave it like you crave the fizz of soda on a hot summer's day. I want you to be ready to fight for your life, not for a while or until the hype settles, but forever! And when the weight starts to come off, I want you to understand it's not over; the fight is for life!

Let us put on our gloves and get ready to RUMBLE!

PEACE,

Dan

Introduction

I'm hungry to lose weight, but most days, I'm just getting by.
~ Journal entry, 2010

I LIKED MYSELF ONCE. It was back when I was 10. Back when I was quick with a joke and full of youthful vigor. Back when being the big kid on the block got you picked first for a game of touch football. When every little boy's dream was to be like Joe Namath, all-star quarterback and the most valuable kid on the block.

Inside those early years of blissful innocence, I dared to dream of such acceptance, a time when nobody stared when I ate more than my share of the food. When no eyes watched with concern, as if I might eat their portion too, and eventually starve off humankind.

"He's a growing boy with a healthy appetite," the adults laughed, elbowing each other with a casual, "boys will be boys."

Those carefree days felt like another man's journey, and I could see every dream abandoned in the front yard of my life. The happiness that once filled my heart was weighed down, literally, by every meal enjoyed when I was not hungry. I looked in a mirror, and I saw

INTRODUCTION

a mound of flesh, an exaggeration of Dan Hawthorne. The real me no longer existed. I was a watered-down version, and my heart was a black hole. Life orbited around me, eyeballing me in complete and utter terror. It, too, feared my darkness.

I was a spectator, trapped inside a self-made Hell.

When one weighs over 650 pounds, it is easy to see yourself as something less than human. The judgment of others feels earned and expected. Most days, I was distracted by more important matters, like the effort it would take to raise my girth off the couch and move down the hallway to the bathroom. Or the array of pain I experienced while attempting to walk, a knife-like sensation cutting at my ankles. And wait until my back registered that it was to hold up my mass! The explicit verbal slurs may have sounded like me, but it was my body screaming in protest.

The pain is just punishment. I deserved and accepted it and would do nothing to make it better. So instead, I merely joined in with mockery, *This is what you get, Dan, for being such a loser!* And I'd continue to taunt as I crossed the room, my weight shifting heavily on a cane for balance.

Aren't you a bit young for a cane, fatty? My alter ego, Beelzebub, relished in a game of self-humiliation. *Look at you. You're pathetic.*

How does a man who once thought of himself as honest and good take up self-loathing as a hobby? I hadn't seen the real me in years. I was not even sure where I put him or if he still existed. My pain was much like my pride, inconsistent and hostile. Every morning when I woke, I choked down those first few moments of discomfort, refusing to leave nirvana for consciousness. Yet, inside, I was living someone else's life, able to forget the integrity of my own. And for a split second, I believed that I could go for a morning run along a beach or put on a pair of normal-sized slacks and take my wife out dancing.

Then I moved, and it hit me; *I am still me.*

Facing my own identity was undoubtedly the first hurdle of every day. And whatever the day brought, I could count on frequent moments of embarrassment. I was choking on my pride as if gagging down a sour pill without the aid of water.

I question was why I bothered to get up at all.

I rarely went anywhere. I didn't venture into view. And if I did, I was with family, at some event where the realization that a chair, unable to hold my mass, awaited me. Words cannot express how it feels when every eye turns to watch, the weight of their cynical gaze seemingly doubling my girth until I'm trudging through the deepest trench to reach my seat.

It was like a game show. *Can he, will he fit?* Everyone waited with bated breath to watch the fat man take a seat.

I knew what they're thinking. *How can someone get that big? Why doesn't he just stop eating? Will the chair even hold him?*

INTRODUCTION

They pondered the horror of it while also questioning and fearing the possibility of it happening to them. I didn't blame others for staring, for judging. I, too, looked at myself and asked, *Who is this sad shell of a man who cannot even tie his shoes?*

For years, the man in the mirror and I had an understanding; my life would be short, and all that was left were the goodbyes. So, in the summer of 2008, my nonverbal farewells began when my family came to visit me, and instead of seeing Danny, the young man with a dream, they saw a vision of slow death. Every facet of my body was swollen, such as fingers that no longer looked like an appendage but rather fleshy sausages with no visible bones.

My mother took one look at my swollen face and concern flooded her eyes. What had happened to Danny, her youngest, her baby? Sadness came from her soul as she watched me struggle to walk, breathe, and function as a human being. My sisters expressed, "We're worried about you, Butch," and the sound of my childhood name brought me to tears.

Unable to face it, I told them what they wanted to hear, "I will get it under control. I will go on a diet." I said anything to convince us all that it was okay.

A lie was more manageable than admitting I would die, that obesity had taken everything, including my self-worth. I smiled in the right moments, said all the words to convince my family they did not have to worry about Danny; they could leave Ocean City and go back to Hagerstown, Maryland, with the confidence that I'd be alright.

Is death what I want? I asked as I stood in the bathroom of a rickety mobile home, lights off, inspecting my reflection. Time passed like a premonition, and I could see not just death but a foreseen agony. Would my heart go first? Would it hurt?

Even in the face of death, addiction called, *Just one cheeseburger, you will be alright.* Beelzebub continued to seduce me, promising me comfort while questioning my existence. *Aren't you one of God's most prized creations? How dare He leave you here with this monster?* I slapped a palm to the mirror, not wanting to see the truth. *Why are others living a whole life while I'm living in shackles?*

Enraged as I was, food controlled me, emotionally and physically. I longed for a taste, that feeling of love just swishing around in my mouth. For when a good meal could mask my shame, give me a sense of peace. But the effects never endured, and reality always crept in; somewhere between a Krumpee's donut and the caramel popcorn on the boardwalk of Ocean City, I'd lost my soul. That once happy-go-lucky kid had fallen into a dark abyss of loneliness, and before I knew it, I was not just that big guy anymore...

I was obese.

Chapter One

Food: The happy times

God is great, God is good, let us thank him for our Jelly Bread.
~ Dinnertime prayer, age eight

Born on June 5th, 1965, to William and Rose Marie Hawthorne, my story begins in a well-adjusted, two-parent, middle-class family. I was loved and nurtured. Every Sunday, we went to church, prayed around the dinner table, and took yearly vacations as a family unit. The youngest of four children, I made good use of all the benefits that came to the unexpected and last Hawthorne-boy-child conceived in the little-big town of Hagerstown, Maryland.

"Danny, turn down the TV. Your father is trying to sleep."

FOOD: THE HAPPY TIMES

Mothers of the 1970s were like magical ninjas—ghosts, appearing from nowhere, with eyes in the back of their heads, forearms like that of a professional pitcher, and able to hurl any object with great accuracy.

"Ah, Mom." My complaint was muffled by soggy Captain Crunch. "It's Saturday."

"Did you hear me?" Her petite frame materialized, eyes bulging like that Wyle E. Coyote character.

"What are you cooking?" I was a master at shifting the topic.

"Slippery pot pie." Her eyes narrowed. "Daniel Wayne, do as I say!"

"Ah, man…" was always a kid's famous last words.

"If Dad gets up, he's going to whip your butt." My brother Billy, the firstborn, sat close by, plotting the action like a football play he could brag to his buddies about later.

I stuck my tongue out, Captain Crunch and all!

"Why don't you turn that TV off, go outside, and get some stink blown off you?" The suggestion was really her final order.

As was typical for an American middle-class family, children were expected to be invisible. Often shooed outside, we ran the streets in packs, like the wild hyenas we had all seen on Mutual of Omaha's *Wild Kingdom* on Sunday night. And with West Virginia five miles to the south and Pennsylvania a mere ten miles to the north, we were unaware that Hagerstown, our playground, was the "Hub City," providing goods and services to Washington, DC. Located between the Blue Ridge and the Allegheny Mountains, in a valley known to locals as Hagerstown Valley, we flourished inside the natural balance of Appalachian down-home hospitality and a hip East-coast spice.

I was a typical kid, preoccupied with Saturday morning cartoons, Big Wheels, and the smash-hit movie *Planet of the Apes*. The historical importance of my hometown, like the fact that the Antietam Battlefield, a Civil War site known as the bloodiest day on American soil, was just up the road, meant little to a boy my age. I was more interested in the latest vinyl album release of my favorite singer, Elvis Presley, than what happened so many years ago.

"Butch, did you take my Flaming Star album again?" my sister Terri, the third in the bunch, shouted from her room adjacent to my own.

I slid the empty record sleeve under my pillow, a mere two seconds before she was standing in my doorway, hands-on-hips, and pointing.

"Why don't you get your own?" She wagged a finger at me.

Get my own? Why would I do that when I have hers?

"It's under his pillow," Crystal, the second-born Hawthorne child, offered, passing behind Terri.

I stuck my tongue out to her too.

Food: The happy times

Pleased with the title as the youngest, I took great joy in these moments of sibling tit-for-tats, and my thoughts rarely roamed outside the radius of my small world. And the best of that world, of Hagerstown itself, was discovered from the seat of my Huffy bicycle. Every inch of the ultra-urban neighborhood was within my grasp.

There was only one thing better than cruising with my friends, one eye on the streetlights—the only curfew any kid acknowledged—and that was the occasional family trip to the department store, on what I called, Saturday-fun-day.

Kresges was the Kmart of the 1970s. And to a boy my age, these outings ranked up there with field games and torturing my sisters. To me, it's easily one of the highlights from my childhood. And though I do not imagine errands with three kids in tow could have been fun for Mom, she never complained. Each trip was unlike the last, and drama would inevitably unfold.

"Now, girls, watch your brother." Mom gave the order, but I was already bent on chaos, and with dimples as big as my 45 inches, I looked cute while doing it.

"Have you seen him?" I heard Crystal whisper to Terri from my covert position.

Like all eight-year-olds, I was virtually invisible when crouched in the center of an overstuffed rack of clothes.

"This is not funny," Terri hissed as I crawled from one rack to another, making a fort on the opposite side.

I watched as both sisters walked to the parallel aisle, flipping shirts and huffing when they found no little brother.

You're getting colder, colder, I silently snickered, then took out a Hot Wheel from my back pocket and settled in for a game of Speed Racer.

While the minutes passed, I ran the toy up my leg and over my knee, plunging it to the carpet with a silent crash. Pushing the car around my back, I paused to listen but heard no girls fussing, no Mom yelling my name. Suspicious, I peeked out from behind a tee-shirt, and seeing it was clear, crawled out on my hands and knees. Even standing at my full height, I still could not see over the garment sleeves, so upon my tippy toes, I went, stretching for a better view.

Nothing, I saw no one. *They left you.* My mind spun like a growing storm, panic rising. Racing up the closest aisle, I passed stacks of cleaning supplies and motor oil, only to find no one, not a soul. *How will I get home?* I wondered as I moped to the front registers.

"Rose Hawthorne, Mrs. Rose Hawthorne, we have your son, Danny, at checkout." The worker-lady held one hand on the microphone and the other on the collar of my shirt.

FOOD: THE HAPPY TIMES

The wait felt like an eternity, but I was thankful when my mom's small frame came around a corner, a frown on her face and two snickering sisters in tow.

"You're not supposed to leave your sisters," my mom reprimanded while the clerk passed me off by the collar like dirty laundry. "Daniel Wayne, what would happen if someone took you?"

All kids my age took this warning in stride; we never found out who that *someone* was, only that, according to our mothers, *someone* was always close by.

"I hope he's the ice cream man," my friends and I would discuss, all agreeing that being kidnapped in a van full of cold treats would be the best.

Though I had lost the battle with my sisters, I had won the war. Because no matter my antics, the outing was always good for junk food and toys!

I can still remember sitting in the cafeteria, at a table for four, bursting with anticipation of those Kresges burgers or the hot roast turkey with yellow gravy. And while Mom and the sisters shuttled food trays from the line to the table, all I could think about were those overly salted fries smothered in ketchup. The meal alone made for a great day, but on this day, something was about to change my world forever.

Set for home, Mom marched me out the storefront, unwittingly passing a gentleman unboxing the newest toy—"The World's Greatest Superhero" Mego action figures. My world shifted on its axis, young eyes scanning over the colorful boxes, neck careening for a better look.

"Mom, look. Mom!" I pulled against the current, needing to see the tiny, blue, yellow, and red-caped figures with names like Superman and Batman.

The toys overflowed the bin, teetering on the edge of the display and emanating a thrill the likes of Christmas morning. The madness, the genius of it all; where had these toys been my whole life? I had to have them.

While sitting shotgun in Dad's blue LTD Ford the whole drive home, I formulated a plan. All eight-year-olds instinctively know how to get what they want and who to get what they want from.

And so, because Dad had us on a tight budget, I knew Mom would be a hard sell. The only question was how to ask her without really asking. Because all kids know, gifts come easier when an adult believes it to be their own idea. So, later that night, while I sat at the family dinner table, chewing happily on my grilled ham and cheese, I executed the plan in my head. Danny's quest for Mego figures, part one.

I imagined my exact words. "Mom, they were less than five dollars!" I'd start with the biggest bang for the buck first—it's cheap.

Then, I'd top it off with young regret. "And I couldn't get them because Dad forgot to give me my allowance." And, if need, I would allow my brown eyes to muster up a few tears.

And just like that, Batman was in my Easter basket, and Robin was given for my birthday. In a blink of an eye, a boyhood bond was formed with the likes of The Dynamic Dual.

It hit me like… Ka-pow!

Later, while I was celebrating my plan with chocolate ice cream, contentment came over me. The world felt right. My thirst for something new was as well-fed as my belly. And I was too young to realize it then, but this moment of true bliss set me on a path, one destined to compare every future moment with this first. The proper ingredients for a happy life were straightforward; all utopian days begin with a new discovery and end with a meal.

Chapter Two

Growing Pains

*Leave him be; he has to pee, let mom-Rosie's
little butchy-beaver be.*
~ Childhood lullaby, age ten

Growing up on Pope Avenue was like living in the middle of a warm family embrace. Back when a neighbor did not think twice about borrowing a cup of sugar. When people knew the names of all the children living in a four-block radius, and they weren't afraid to reprimand any number of kids, should the need arise. And it often did.

My grandmother (Nan) and Aunt Thelma (her sister-in-law) lived a few blocks away from my family home. Some kids are lucky to have two grandmothers, but it felt like I had three thanks to my aunt's undying admiration for little-o'-me. Aunt Thelma never had any children of her own, and other than her cats, she took an extra shine to me.

Every day, I would ride my bike down to the end of Pope Avenue to check in on Nan, secretly hoping that she would send me to the local store for a quick this-or-that.

"Nan. Nan!" I hollered, dropping my Huffy to her front stoop, and entering the home without a knock.

"Daniel Wayne, don't let your aunt's kitten out." My grandmother hurried from the kitchen, a red apron flapping around her knees.

I snatched the white bundle up without missing a beat. "I came to see if you needed anything from Hull's?" Like all neighborhood corner stores, Hull's was a gathering place for gossip and basic home needs, like bread and milk. But to us kids, it was the daily stop for sweets.

"I need a gallon of milk." She reached into her apron's pocket, adding a polite epitaph, "If you're going that way, that is?"

I am always going that way. I smirked as she dropped three dollars into my palm. But then, I did the math. Milk was a buck-fifty, which meant I had...enough for 20 tootsie rolls, a Shenandoah chocolate milk and a cherry pie!

Even in those early days, I planned my day around food. If Mother set the family table around 5:30 PM, just in time for my father's arrival home, then I knew if I went to Nan's around 3:30 PM, I could score a pre-dinner treat. It was not unusual for me to have a taste of Nan's dinner and then rush to my aunt's and try some of her homemade chocolate peanut butter fudge, all before dinner at my own home. And because I was Aunt Thelma's boy, if nothing were prepared and ready when I got there, all I had to do was ask, and beautiful smells would begin.

"Danny, patience is the key to fudge," Aunt Thelma explained, her dark blonde hair rolled into a neat bun, with cat-like reading glasses teetering on the bridge of her nose.

I can still see her now, hovering over a glass bowl, allowing me to lick the spoon while instructing when to drop the tiny dab of wet fudge into the water. If it stayed in a ball, it was ready.

Man-o-man, the anticipation would build while waiting for that chocolaty sweetness to set; it was almost too much for a young boy to take! And when it was time, I would grab myself a cold glass of milk and go to town. If allowed, I could eat a whole plate, no problem, and then get back on my bike and arrive home just in time for dinner with the family.

Two dinners in one day, what a great gig!

My childhood reads like the whose-who of comfort foods; if I received good marks in school, Aunt Thelma would whip me up a batch of her homemade chocolate cookies. If I ran an errand for my grandmother, Nan,

I would sweetly ask for brownies to be waiting for me when I returned. And because my family loved to eat, celebrating every triumph with food was ordinary.

It is Christmas, let's eat! It is somebody's birthday, more food.

And on Sundays, at the Evangelistic Temple, the after-service event was often lined with Mom, Nan, and Thelma's specialty dishes. Of course, all my favorite foods were available, like Mom's fried chicken or Nan's moist meatloaf and baked beans.

The evangelistic way fascinated me, and I watched curiously as members of the congregation fell into the aisles, as the adults explained, drunk in the spirit and speaking in a tongue that I had never heard before. But nothing confused me more than the day I witnessed a baptismal celebration along the edge of a river when a local woman stepped into the muddy waters for Jesus.

What did dirty water have to do with God? I just could not figure it. But later that day, back at Aunt Thelma's, while supervising three white rescue kitties, I had an idea. Lifting one of the cats, I dunked its back two paws into a bucket of brown rainwater, proclaiming at the top of my voice, "I now baptize thee in the name of Jesus!" And then repeated the ritual until all three cats waddled around the yard, half white and half brown.

"Daniel Wayne, why are my kittens brown?" Thelma was continuously checking on me because *quiet boys are naughty boys.*

"I baptized them in the bucket," I proudly proclaimed, and even minus a tooth, my grin was full.

"Oh, my," she placed a hand to her cheek.

"They can see Jesus now, right?"

"Well, honey, let's go inside and talk about this over pie."

And just like that, I was eating, again!

Though the Hawthornes ate well, my parents scrimped to feed us. For even in 1975, food for a family of six was costly. So my mother cooked simple dishes, considered poor people's delight, like butter beans spread over toast. And while my father worked long days, commuting to DC in the wee hours of the morning, my mother kept busy tending to her four kids.

While most of my friends' mothers did not work outside the home, Mom applied for seasonal work over the summer when kids were out of school and often away on sleepovers at friends' places or bible camp. Upon our return, food was the topic at the next home meal. What did you eat? Did you like it? If we had an out-of-town guest, my parents took great care when deciding which local restaurant would represent Hagerstown best. It was necessary not just to explain the difference between a Sloppy Joe, where onions and green peppers are present, and a Steamer, where they are not, but show the dish firsthand. Marylanders, in general, like to eat; it is a sub, not a hoagie, slipper pot pie, and not dumplings. If you are a food lover, then Maryland is a beautiful place to grow up, and as it happened for me, expand out.

***

By middle school, I had a set of friends that ranged from the popular to misfits. The cute girls befriended me because I was chunky-sweet, like a candy bar, and mostly harmless. The popular boys tolerated me, much like a king would a court jester; I made a dull day tolerable. But the bulk of my friends were the kids in between, the ones the popular kids mostly did not see, the ones that prayed they would make it to 12th grade with as few scars as possible.

The school was not my favorite place, but I earned my fair share of Bs and Cs. I was already bigger than most of my classmates, but I hung to the fact that the adults said I was "big-boned," which made it okay. But like most kids in their early teens, my confidence was putty, soft, and bendable, and I relied on friends to help boost my ego.

"Do it, do it," urged Dave while I waved the sharp end of a pencil closer and closer to Mrs. Snyder's posterior. Now, I do not know whether she stepped back into the tip, or I voluntarily poked her, but she got a goose, and I went to the office.

Well-liked amongst my peers, humor was my way of coping with the reality of looking different. Being the funny guy was way better than being that chunky kid who will not take his shirt off in the boy's locker room or refuses to be skins—no matter how much the shirts team sucked! I was naturally artistic, which I channeled by drawing cartoons of teachers with my friend, Less, who's now a graphic illustrator.

I'd come to find out that teachers do not appreciate being the subject of student artwork! So yeah, I went to the office for that one, too.

My friends and I did all the usual things teenagers do, like dirtball fights and midnight movies at Long Meadow Cinema. We must have seen *Dawn of the Dead* twenty times. And in our teen fantasies, we were the original lost boys, and Hagerstown was ours for the taking. And the world had not stepped in to echo our limitations, so we didn't think we had any.

The great thing about being young is that we are not yet aware of our shortcomings, like being too tall, or the imperfections of one's complexion, until an unthinking senior classmate tells us. It seems that we are born to love others and ourselves from childhood, and it is not until hormones rage that we begin to listen to the negative whispers of others.

"Come here, dough-boy!" The senior was a football player, full of muscles. "Lie down and take it like a man, Hawthorne."

It was freshman hazing time, and I had been waiting my turn.

Unfortunately, because I was a good size, I took my father's advice and tried out for South High's freshman football team, drawing unwanted attention. I was like a six-point buck to a Senior Varsity predator.

"I gotcha." I felt his hand touch my shoulder, and I melted to the ground. I rolled over and offered him my soft underbelly, already knowing what was going to happen; I had seen it done to two of my friends the week prior.

"Don't fight," he huffed, hovering over me and yanking up my shirt to expose my rolls. "Well, look what we have here, a real heifer."

More seniors circled like vultures to roadkill.

I could have fought one; it is not like I was weak. But outnumbered, I figured it was just my turn, and the freshman before me had managed to survive, so I turned my head and gave way to the boy, pinching and poking until my soft belly became a bright red. The pain was deep, and my skin burned, much like my pride. But as fast as it had started, it was over.

When the sturdy boy rolled off me, he took a moment to laugh over his handy work. Then said, "Lord, Hawthorne, eat fewer donuts, man!" And just like that, the pack ran off in search of more newcomers.

15 was an awkward age, and while most of my friends sat in class, distracted by girls and Ms. Pac-Man, I was dreaming about—you guessed it—LUNCH. That coveted school time break, when hundreds of

kids rush like cows to the trough, compelled to eat up whatever slop is given. I would watch the clock, already mulling over my food order.

Was I going to have a cold or hot plate, milkshake or chocolate milk?

Remember the yellow gravy? Even a non-foodie remembers that somewhat scary and yet somehow coveted high school gravy. Though its over-processed consistency, no doubt, has given many children from the 1970s and 80s some form of adult disease, it was a delight!

One either hated it or loved it. Take a guess which one I was?

There was not much I hated where school food was concerned. The lunchroom was my comfort zone. Not only did I eat until I was loaded, but fueled by the latest lunchtime poison, I flexed my mischievous nature. I dared my friends to do whatever I fancied, like when I paid Richard to walk around with mash potatoes and peas on his freshly shaved head. We all laughed like crazy, and then I felt guilty, not for bribing Richard to do it, but for wasting good mash potatoes and peas!

I was too young to see a problem brewing, but I did notice my friends could care less what was on the school menu. Where I counted the seconds to the food bell, my friends turned up their noses to the school's chef.

"How can you eat that?" John scrunched his nose. "It looks like the crap inside my baby brother's diapers!"

I turned up a spoon of poop and flicked it his way, and while everyone laughed, I once again had used humor to avoid a food debate. Because of being funny, loud, and slightly daring, my worries about being different disappeared.

My prankster persona was not limited to school, and from an early age, my dream to become a radio broadcaster flourished in my childhood home. But, unfortunately, the goal disrupted my family, as I practiced for the day when I would go live on the air, secretly taping family conversations around the house, even the disputes. Then later, I would record my voice, providing commentary to these verbal interchanges, only to replay them to my horrified parents.

"Welcome to candid-tape with Dan Hawthorne. Here's the latest dispute between Mom and Dad." And when they realized I had captured sensitive adult moments, the reprimand, including an embarrassing explanation, just did not seem worth it.

Score: kid one, parents zero.

At some point, I mastered the art of voices. "Billy, William David," I mimicked my father, "tell that girl to stop calling the house."

"Why don't you tell her?" I echoed back, now in my brother's voice, and then ducked behind the couch, waiting for a parental unit to make an appearance. And when Dad arrived, not Mom, I made a quick exit on my hands and knees.

"Rosie?" I heard him call for my mother because we all looked to Mom for answers when anything was off.

My favorite stunt was to call home from a friend's house and leave dinner requests in my father's voice. "Rosie, can you make some bean soup? It's been a tough day." Now, bean soup was my favorite, but my father's was roast beef.

To this day, I wonder whether Mom knew it was me calling. And did she simply decide to accommodate my request? Or maybe, she was just too busy running a household to waste time confronting the details? I mean, she was going to cook a full meal for a party of six, no matter the day of the week, so what differenced did the meal itself make?

Either way, from my young perspective, it was all in a day's work as a growing artist, and I was going to be a radio GOD. So I needed a lot of practice. And if I managed to score bean soup along the way, all the better!

Chapter Three

Love and Radio

This is Dan Kelly in the air-chair. Welcome to my weekend gig. Give me a call at 797-7303. That's your direct line to my big behind.
~ **Words from a radio God, 1987**

I WAS NOT LUCKY IN love, but in the late-1980s, friends considered me fortunate. New opportunities seemingly materialized, like how my radio dream came true one night at a party when I dialed the request line at WQCM radio station.

"Yeah, this is the Big E calling from rock-n-roll heaven." Mimicking my hero, Elvis Presley, I was careful to stutter in all the right places, "I-I was hoping y'all play me a special song. I'm lonesome, missing my Cilla tonight."

Soon, Burning Love blared through the party-house, and we all danced like crazy, everyone amazed with the big guy who would do anything for a laugh. And when the song was over, I heard the same DJ ask, "Whoever just called in as Elvis, call me back," and in doing so, I landed a job interview that next day.

My on-air name was Dan Kelley, and as Dan Kelly, I could be any shape of a man! Girls thought I had a sexy voice, but I did not discover this until my first remote radio gig, when girls appeared more interested in me than my thick sides.

"Do you have a girlfriend?" a female listener purred by my side while my older and wiser partner chuckled close by.

We had been broadcasting live on location for a mere thirty minutes, and suddenly, I found myself in the throes of female infatuation.

"Would you like to apply for the job?" the coworker asked on my behalf.

"No, no." I panicked like in middle school when accused of crushing on Mrs. Scott, the older but very gorgeous art teacher. "No really, no offense, but no."

While the attention of young women came with the job, and my male friends envied me, urging me to use this newfound power for their benefit if not for myself, I lacked the confidence. In my mind, I was still the big kid that didn't get the girl. And even when I allowed my ego to escalate, I would inevitably do or say something stupid and come crashing back to earth. Like the time I tried to impress a cute redhead that worked at the local convenience store.

"Hello, Kimberly." I noted her name tag. "Did you pick the store's music?"

She looked at me, puzzled, so I pointed upward to the sound of Michael Jackson's *Billie Jean* filtering through the store.

"Uh, no," she said, shifting nervously.

"I'm only teasing. I like your choice in radio stations," I said, trying to salvage my dreadful attempt at flirting. "I work at WQCM."

She looked me up and down, eyes widening from a sudden realization. "I know you! You're that late-night guy with the funny voices."

"Yeah, that's me." I rolled my eyes, as if to imply the job was a bore. "Hey, what's your favorite song?"

Offering to spin a tune was fun, and I did it a lot, taking names from random retail workers—girls and boys—and then dedicating the songs to them later that night. On that day, Kimberly's name went into my pocket, but her phone number did not. I did not ask her on a date because that would require the real Dan to step up, and I preferred to hide behind my role as radio jock.

"That's right, folks, Michael Jackson is sold out. Congrats to those that scored tickets," I bantered. "Now here's one for Kimberly, working hard at the mini-mart; it may not be the King of Pop, but it's Bon Jovi, the King of Hair, and Living on a Prayer."

I pushed the microphone away, clicked the audio to the off position, and looked to my coworker, who was grabbing his jacket to leave.

"Todd, man, you should see the redhead down at the mini-mart!" Todd was married, but I kept talking. "She is so pretty I would drink her bathwater."

Todd turned, half-humored, his eyes flashing to the soundboard. "Dan, your microphone is hot."

"Oh shit!" I spun in my seat, and, seeing my mistake, flipped the microphone fully into the off position.

"And now, you've cursed over the air too." He was laughing, and while on his way out, added, "Don't burn the place down, son, but if you do, don't call me."

I avoided that store for weeks, afraid that Kimberly heard my blunder on the air. But Hagerstown is small, and there are only so many places to get my favorite chocolate milk, so eventually, I had to go back. And as luck would have it, she was standing behind the counter, smiling as I came forward.

"I heard you." She covered a laugh with her hand.

"I'm sorry you heard that." I handed her a dollar.

"I'm not," she said, hesitating before taking my money. "It was funny!"

"Well, I'm glad someone thought so." I picked up my milk and made a quick exit without her phone number, yet again!

The Giant in Me

I was never Don Juan, a player-of-women; I just wanted a good girl. I did not want a fling. I wanted a girl to love and respect forever.

Renee was her name. She had red hair, and on the petite side, she made my 5'10 seem tall, and my 350-pound frame felt right when standing next to her. And from the sidelines of a party, I watched her, gaging her sense of fun. She came with a friend, Gale, who came with my best buddy, Jimmy. Gale and Jimmy had been dating, and Renee was one of her younger cousins.

The Budget Inn on the dual highway was party central for my gang of friends. Someone would rent a room, and we'd fill the tub with beer, spin music, and laugh until morning. Compared to the mischief of today, it was innocent fun that felt reckless at the time. Mostly because some of us were old enough to drink and some were not—bottom line, nobody cared if you were 19 or 21.

When it was my turn to rent the room, I arrived early to set up the beer and food. Room 215 was assigned at check in, and the first order of business was to call all my friends and announce where the party would be located. Looking back, I realize how nice it would have been to have the technology of today—the ability to text instead of dialing each friend, one by one.

The minute I pushed open the room door, hands full of beer, a feeling of dread greeted me. The hairs on my forearms stood straight up as if charged by electrostatic. The air felt dangerous, sparked by something negative. And the dark energy was so thick, my stomach began to turn.

I had felt this sense of dread before, something terrible had happened in this room. And with every fiber in my body, I believed it to be true. So, I marched back down to the front desk, beer still in hand. And while waiting to speak my peace, I scanned my memory; what had happened here? Had I heard something in the news? And by the time the hotel clerk stepped behind the lobby desk, I had it.

"Excuse me." I politely flagged the same young lady from before. "I'm sorry to bother you, but is 215 the room where that man had killed himself in last week?"

Her eyes went wide. Her blank expression told me all I needed to know.

"Something bad happened in that room. I cannot stay in there tonight…" I was working my way towards asking for another room when she interrupted me.

"I'm sorry, we've been given orders not to talk about that."

"I understand," I told her, then went on to explain how I can feel the energy of that room. How I'm sensitive to human vitality. And she did what all people do when I tell them I can feel ghosts. She dropped her eyes, straightened her shoulders, and went to the task of getting me another room. No questions asked.

Her reaction didn't surprise me; it's precisely why I don't talk about this gift, or curse, depending on one's views. And I find, typically, it's the latter, as people think "I can see dead people," or that "red-rum" is scribbled in red on my back! None of it is true. What I feel is merely a body reaction—my hairs stand up, my stomach turns, a cold draft runs over me.

To be honest, most structures give off energy. And it's not always bad, but on this night, it was terrible. Whatever had happened in that room was dark, and so, the party moved to room 315; one floor up and clean of bad mojo!

And when young men throw a party, in a small town like Hagerstown, girls will inevitably come. No male needs to spread the word; it's the call of the wild. Young souls are immediately drawn to other young souls having fun. So, the tiny hotel room was soon packed with way more fun than it really could hold, but nobody cared.

I barely even noticed the crowd. I was busy getting to know Renee. Immediately, I was drawn to her innocence and vulnerability, the way she didn't get the joke or how she knew something was different about me but couldn't quite place it.

"So, are you the voice of Elvis-P on WQCM?"

Mimicking the King had gotten me not only a job but a guest spot during the afternoon drive time hour. Listeners loved the character, and to make it more fun, no one knew the identity behind the voice. It was a station secret. And like all the young adults in the area, Renee tuned in for the Top 40 hits and the mystery.

"Maybe it is." I smiled coyly, going for cute and not arrogant. "But maybe not."

Not a big drinker, I sat there watching and laughing with Renee as the others got drunk. It's not that I did not want to join the fun, but, because I was a big guy, it took crazy amounts of alcohol to get a buzz, so I rarely tried.

Though Renee did not have much to say, and I've always been a talker, we enjoyed each other's company. An innocence emanated that made me want to protect her, from life, from the other wolves in the crowd. But our relationship did not spark with what some might call love-at-first-sight. Still, in the months that followed, we had the kind of fun that the young understand—reckless and unrestrained, driving to Ocean City in the summers and riding motorbikes through the Maryland hills in the fall.

My greatest memories of that time came when Jimmy and II had bought our first motorcycles. He would get Gale, Renee, and I together then off we'd go, racing through the cornfields of Maryland, a smell of damp wheatgrass in the air.

"I need to use the bathroom," I shouted to Renee, who was snuggled up behind me on my blue Honda 500. I felt her nod in agreement along my back.

Waving to Jimmy, we pulled up to Hardy's hamburger joint, somewhere in Pennsylvania, and parked.

"Can I have the keys?" Renee asked, interrupting my stretch.

And standing upright, I turned to look at her, wondering what she was all about. Then, after a moment of consideration, I tossed the key her way.

Inside, as we all enjoyed our burger and fries, my mind returned to the key she had nestled in her pocket. "Renee, why do you need my bike key?

Focused on the food, she spoke in a low tone. "So you won't leave me here," she said, time seemingly impeded by the admission.

I looked to Gale, who merely shrugged. "Has someone done this to you before?"

"Yes." Renee took a fry, examined it as if deciding whether to elaborate and then brought it to her mouth with an end-of-story finality.

I was young, but I recognized the fragility of a woman who honestly believed I might get on my bike and leave. An urge swelled inside of me, a desire to prove to Renee that she could trust me. I vowed to show her I was different, that my heart would never allow me to treat anyone in such a manner, especially not a vulnerable young woman such as herself.

Three months later, I asked Renee to move in with my parents on Pope Avenue. Unfortunately, after 'the key' incident, I became privy to the fact that Renee was discontent, and did not feel safe where she resided, so I could not sit back and do nothing—thankfully, my parents agreed.

As mature as I felt, I did not see myself as a provider, a father, or a lifetime partner at 23. I was still collecting Mego action figures, drinking beer with the boys, and spinning records part-time over a broadcast channel. I was not thinking about anything that might involve making a home with someone. But after pressure from both of our families to 'make things right', Renee and I were married that fall.

It was a small affair, just family. We all gathered at the justice of the peace. And with everyone hovering about, waiting for our turn, I paced the room. Deep inside, a small voice rattled my nerves.

Are you sure you want this? Is she really the one? It played like a broken record.

As my nerves escalated, I watched my mother, wondering if I'd ever seen her happier. Her baby boy was about to tie the knot, and she was counting the minutes until a court official would come through those metal doors and call us up.

"You okay, Son?" My father slapped my back, interrupting the fretting and nail-biting. "You know you don't have to do this."

Now, he tells me. Of course, I must do this. I asked her, she said yes! And look at my mother. There was no way I was going to ruin this because I got cold feet.

The Giant in Me

"I'm fine. We're going to be fine," were my famous last words.

At the start, we rarely considered the future, did not care where we lived, whether we owned or rented a home. So who was going to lead this crazy union anyway—me? The man who believed eating food should be an Olympic sport and thought life as a romantic movie? Or the girl who had been told horrible lies by trusted adults, and therefore, trusted no one?

Life was a struggle for Renee and me; right from the start, troubled finances loomed around every corner. It turns out Radio Gods do not make much money, and frankly, Renee grew frustrated with our lifestyle, or lack thereof. In addition, she disliked my Disc Jockey career, which cultivated female attention, none of which I invited.

The entry-level position did not pay well, typical of an industry where time behind a microphone is what gets one ahead. And while Renee worked a full-time job herself, it still wasn't enough. So, I took on a second job to supplement our household, further limiting my time at home. Unfortunately, this schedule put a strain on our relationship, and Renee began to resent the career that I loved.

"Why can't you get a regular 9 to 5 job?"

We had gone over this a million times before—radio versus a standard job—and every time my heart would feel pulled in two directions. "It won't always be like this, Renee. I just need to put in the time, and the perks will come."

When the stress would heat up, I turned to food for comfort. I could quickly obtain anything I wanted over the air because when you are a DJ on a Top40 station, "Man-o-man, I can go for a nice cold glass of chocolate milk right now," was all I had to say before Madonna's, *Like a Virgin* blared over the airwaves. And before long, someone would be knocking on the door of the studio, chocolate milk in hand!

I ordered pizzas, donuts, cakes, chocolates; everything yummy was on the table.

At one point, I even made up a game called "Begging for Food," where my radio partner or I would call a favorite eatery in town. We would tell them we're on-the-air, and then start complimenting menu items we genuinely enjoyed. The idea was that the business would get free radio advertisement, and in turn, they would send us over those items we just told them we loved.

I ate my way through the '90s!

Our first year of marriage went by fast; we raced through the weeks until the months had passed into years, and neither could remember where the time had gone or recite one thing we had accomplished together. Well into our third year, we were already going through the motions, and other than the gold band on our fingers, we had little in common.

I liked deep conversations. The longer, the better. Renee did not. She loved reality television, heated drama like Jerry Springer, anything with troubling stories and dissolving relationships, which made me crazy. I loved Elvis. She tolerated him. I believed in God and the spiritual life. She believed in only what she could see. But we were married, so as most couples do, we forged on, and the years fell away like a falling house of cards—a random mess.

Chapter Four

Home at the bottom

I would not wish this on my worst enemy.
~ Journal entry, 2010

It's with great sadness that we inform you; severance letters always start with regret—we hate to let you go, but we are anyway. Then end with an explanation that inevitably would state the cause was a change of musical format.

Great. I tossed the paper to the tabletop by my side and clicked off the lamplight. The room was completely black; not even a streetlight from outside dared to interrupt the mood. Three stations in the last three years, that's how many had either closed or changed format, no longer needing a man behind the microphone.

What am I going to tell Renee? The idea of explaining my, yet again, lack of employment had my stomach in an uproar.

I want a milkshake. Though better judgement growled a warning, I was out the door and under the golden arches within minutes. While waiting, Beelzebub provoked, *You need to feel better, and food always makes you feel better.*

Somehow this reasoning made sense, and before I could work it out, a voice asked in the night, "Hello, welcome to… can I take your order?"

Without a thought, I answered, "I'll take two cheeseburgers, a large fry, a large milkshake, an apple pie, and a Coke."

Every item held a hope that halfway through the milkshake, or maybe the cola, I would feel better. And while parked under a shattered streetlight, I ate every bite and raced to the relief I expected to find at the finish line.

Bite. Chew. Swallow. Repeat. Repeat. Repeat and gone.

My stomach gurgled from the insult. One might think that I would enjoy the after emotions, like a cigarette after sex. But self-hate moves fast; a swell of guilt bursts, and ultimately comes the last-ditch effort to make it all better, like buying a new car, or in this case, the idea to move three hundred miles to the town of Ocean City, Maryland.

Though I had expected Renee to reject the idea, I was happy when she agreed, suggesting the beach could fix our problems. Like most Marylanders, she had romantic ideals about beach life. And even though my weight had escalated well into the 400s, we talked about walks on the beach, as if I could, or we even would, like the salt air would miraculously give us a second chance.

Mostly, I was counting on a change of scenery to invigorate our life together. "This can be a new start, Renee." I glanced over, trying to read her thoughts while the miles passed out the car's window.

"We can get healthy, walk the beach every day." I paused when her eyes snapped to me.

"How are *you* going to walk?" Her tone was double-edged, accusing, and judgmental.

"I *can* lose the weight. I just need to keep junk foods out of the house."

"What am I going to eat?"

Our life did not consist of gourmet meals; we had pallets like that of teenagers.

"I'll do the cooking," I tried. "We can eat chicken and salads."

"I don't eat that."

"I know, but it wouldn't hurt to try."

Look at you, groveling like a baby, echoed Beelzebub.

"Let's just try, Renee, please?"

She thought about this. "Fine. But you're doing everything."

"Not a problem. I'll even cook."

When we left Hagerstown, I told myself that it was fate. My friend and fellow radio enthusiast, Sam, was already down there and had us set up to do a Saturday night show like we had done in Hagerstown years before. And once I was back to work, it was not long before Renee and I had slipped into the resort lifestyle, meeting friends every Thursday night at the Harbor Side Bar for their steamed shrimp special and a cold brew. Then on Fridays, we would hit one of the many crab houses, and Saturday was our night for Dover Downs or Herrington slots.

So much for salad, fatty, Beelzebub prompted.

Radio was no more dependable in Ocean City than in Hagerstown, and soon, I applied for a job at a large retailer.

"Alright, all you happy workers, rally around," the shift boss spoke in an enthusiastic voice. "What are we going to do today?"

"Make customers happy!" everyone but me yelled back.

"And how are we going to do it?"

"Safely!"

To take a creative soul like me and box them in with corporate nonsense should be listed as a crime. It was no wonder to me that a painter would choose to create art along the edge of a river, living on pennies, rather than sacrifice the creativity that gave them their very breath. My true self was dying with every passing hour spent inside this vortex of merchandize Hell, and after a few more years, my weight climbed to a morbid size.

I was in a vicious cycle of striving to be happy, not finding happiness, and then trying to eat my way out from the lack of joy—while still not seeing any happiness.

For more than eight years, Renee and I had been living inside this coastal town, encircled within its beauty, from the glassy, slick bay waters on the West side of Ocean City's peninsula to the thrashing sea at the East. There was so much beauty to soak in, and yet the essence was lost to me. I was as hard as the driftwood that littered the deep coastline.

Sure, my coworkers inside the halls of retail Hell loved me. I was seemingly a happy worker. My friends did not see my emotional suffering; they only saw the jolly Dan-face I put on every day for everyone. But darkness, fueled by regret and hopelessness, grew with every minute of each day, and there was no relief from it, except when I was eating. And by the summer of 2010, my life had become a reality TV show.

"Hey, Dan, you're sure looking good." Bob, my neighbor, waved to me from the edge of our adjacent yards.

It surprises me how often people feel it is acceptable to comment on someone's body size and how often they get it wrong! I was now 500 pounds. How can anyone 'look good?'

"Thank you, Bob. I'm trying."

Liar, all you are striving for is an all-you-can-eat buffet. Beelzebub missed nothing.

"But it's not easy, buddy," I said, feeling the weight of my honesty.

"You know, son…" Because Bob was in his 70's, the title warmed me. "There's something I've been meaning to talk to you about."

I locked my knees, pushed my shoulders back, and steadied myself.

"You know, it's none of my business, but…"

"Go on," I encouraged.

"Well, I had to consider…"

"What is it, Bob?" *Just say it, already,* I internally screamed.

"Dan, after you leave the house, a man comes over. He stays a little over an hour, and then he leaves."

There it was, Bob's troubling secret.

"And how often does this happen?"

What difference does that make, idiot? Beelzebub heckled from the front row of my consciousness.

"Ah, it doesn't matter…" I waved him off. "But thanks for telling me, I sure appreciate it." Then,

I turned for the house, letting Bob off the hook while allowing myself some final dignity.

"Oh, good!" Bob's relief echoed from behind. "Very well then…"

When I arrived at my front door, feeling emotionally numb, I settled onto a porch chair. While Bob quickly retreated to his house, I watched an orange sun slip below the horizon. Usually, I would have picked Renee up from work, but earlier that day, she had called and told me she had a ride.

What now? I felt conflicted. *Do I go and pick her up anyway? Maybe I do nothing? Do I even care?*

As the next hour crept by, the smell from the Italian sauce I had put on the stove earlier wafted around me. Our fur kids, three cats in all, gathered around the windows, watching me with great interest and concern. My mind was blank; I was simply waiting. And finally, when a white van rolled down our street, a mix of dread and excitement filtered through me, like a pressure valve finally releasing. I sank further in my seat, my large frame obstructed by the home's white porch columns. The van slowly rolled past, coming to a stop a few houses up, and thankfully, out of Bob's sight. Break lights flickered as the vehicle set to park, and then all went dark.

While I watched the van, the cats watched me, a group effort in assessing the situation. *I should be mad, should I not?* I turned and looked at the oldest feline in our fur family, who merely blinked back an answer. *Yeah, I don't know what's going on either.*

The night was hot for Maryland, and while I waited, the sweat dripped down my back while fireflies blinked around my face. *I like fireflies.* The thought flickered as my gaze alternated between the bugs and the vehicle parked up the street.

45 minutes. That's how long it took before my wife stepped out of this unknown person's van and walked towards the house. The wrongness of it peaked when the vehicle suddenly made a U-turn, and a man's profile came into view. While his features were cloaked in the night, he slowed to examine my figure in the shadows and then made a quick exit.

"Did you have a good day?" I asked, chuckling over the absurd situation.

My laughter gave away my covert position, and Renee startled to a stop on the first step.

"What are you doing out here?" Her tone was clipped, just the everyday life of an unhappy wife.

"I'm finally understanding," I said as she took the last step onto the porch.

Her eyes burned over me, a laser in the darkness. Time slowed, and our silence took on a presence, like an uninvited spectator — a juror sent to judge this sad trial. When Renee turned to enter the house, muttering something about food and hunger, a gavel fell. The verdict was in; we were over.

***

"They just need to reach the bottom." We have all heard the saying. The idea is excellent, but sadly, "the bottom" does not come and announce itself; it sneaks in and sets up shop under our noses. So even while it was redecorating, changing the feng shui of the room, I focused on everything but "the bottom."

I blamed life. Then I blamed God, everyone, and anyone for my troubles. Even Renee was tiptoeing around the unhappy giant in the room. And when she was home, we would fight, never agreeing nor even listening to the other's valid complaints, voices raised in indignation and self-proclaimed injustice.

No, it takes a while to recognize the bottom for what it is—a wake-up call.

The other misconception of life at "the bottom" is that people seem to believe that once we arrive there, we suddenly see the error of our ways, and the revelation makes us pick up camp and run for the brighter side of life. They do not realize we have unpacked a lot of crap here at the bottom. We are not sure we want to leave it behind. I mean, there may be a big waste of life hanging around down here, but it is our life. And we believe it's all we have.

My wake-up alarm rang on many fronts. My blood pressure and cholesterol were off the charts. Now over 600 pounds, I was forced to leave my retail job due to mobility problems and remained unemployed. And with no pressing appointments, I was free to do as I pleased. Each morning, after taking Renee to work, I would stop for my breakfast and order not just one but two sausage, egg, and cheese biscuits, hash browns, and a large coffee. As was routine, I would have chocolate milk or some other sweet to enjoy as a treat. And while I was consuming what was essentially breakfast number two, I was thinking about the next food fix and where to obtain it.

I was comfortable at "the bottom." By now, food controlled me; it set the tone for the day and the pace of each evening. It was as powerful as any drug or alcohol I could have consumed. Addicts will tell you they need it. And my body did need it; of this fact, I am sure.

I could be cruising the streets, window down, and smell the many buffets and food havens. Instantly, that would set my mind on food, and before I knew it, I was picking up my four-piece fried chicken from English's Diner or my tacos from one of the many Latin restaurants.

Eating felt good. The taste, the imagined love, swishing around in my mouth, took me away from my shame and embarrassment. Food comforted me. I felt satisfied for the few moments it took to consume it. The fried chicken took me back to Nan's house, meatloaf back to the family dinners at 5 PM with Dad.

Was I hungry? Did I need to eat? No. But I needed the comfort my friend food could bring me. I had a botched life, had failed as a husband and a provider. By now, "the bottom" had become home. And I defended it like anyone would when threatened.

If others can eat all they want, you can too, Beelzebub and I agreed.

I would see healthy people eating ice cream and tasty pizza and tell myself, *Hey, they look healthy.* I convinced myself no harm could come from a few bad food choices. And as I became less and less mobile, it became harder to bandage the feelings of a non-achiever. The more I sat dormant, the more I ate to escape, the more weight I gained, 500 and then 600, until the summer of 2010, my weight had climbed to 650 pounds.

My feet never touched the sand. I never walked the boardwalk, and soon, I never walked at all. I turned down invites to bonfires and parties. Renee and I became secluded because I did not want to be seen by anyone. A few friends tried to reach into my life at "the bottom," but how could they help me? What could they possibly say that I had not heard before?

"Dan, I'm worried about you," was typically the go-to expression, because frankly, they were speechless! They could not believe what they saw, and I could not explain. So we were two confused people, one grasping for helpful words while the other was adding up the weight gained since the last visit.

What they say is true. It is lonely at the bottom.

CHAPTER FIVE

GET REAL

Nobody cares if I exist.
~ Journal entry, 2010

I HELD MYSELF RESPONSIBLE FOR my obesity. However, *God has abandoned you, left you to die,* and *he does not care,* was always a good backup whenever blaming myself got old. And in my hour of need, crippled by fear, I lacked the courage to ask for help.

"Thank you for tying my laces," I said, feeling less like a man than ever before.

Renee simply grunted over the task.

At 650 pounds, I no longer slept in a bed. Instead, I napped, upright in the living room recliner, sad and fearful of asphyxia. While an irreconcilable difference separated Renee and I, my obesity had left us utterly alone. We were trapped inside the grips of codependency. When Renee looked at me, she took comfort in what was familiar, a husband in title alone. And when I saw my wife, I saw what I believed was the only woman in the world who would accept the giant I'd become.

"I'm guessing tying my shoes wasn't what you had in mind when we married?" A lot can be implied in a joke.

Her hand stilled. Then, with a tug, she finished the knot, and in looking up to me, I saw a mix of emotions in her eyes — regret, sadness, fear, and uncertainty.

"Not exactly, no," Renee said pointedly, then got up and headed to the door. "I don't know what I expected, but it wasn't this."

"I imagine not."

If Renee and I were anything, we were persistent. Our phycological reliance was approaching a 15-year benchmark.

"I'm going to be late," she said without looking back.

The roles switched; Renee now worked as a cook at a local steak house, while I played housewife. And despite our problems, I drew Renee's nightly baths, lighting candles at the end of the workday. But, honestly, there was no making up for her disappointment, and in thinking back to those niceties and her eyeballing me like I had gone mad, one can only laugh.

Just lose weight already. Get a job, Beelzebub echoed what everybody in the room was thinking.

But I did not lose weight, no job was in my future, and as the finance strings continued to tighten, we took in a renter. Tommy was in his early 20s. And Tommy had a sexual lifestyle that we knew nothing about until Asian porn blared from his room at all hours of the night!

"What in the Hell is that?" Renee stomped into the living room, marching over to where I sat awake in my big-boy chair.

"Sounds like porn." I stated the obvious, folding my arms under the back of my head, amazed at my life.

Why not porn? The revelation, the wickedness, felt like a wrong-way turndown Damnation Avenue on my way to Hell. *I'm already going that way. What's one more moral insult?*

First, I had wrongly expected a change of scenery to heal our marriage, and second, I had given up on life. We were all racing to a metal-crashing end. It was just a matter of who was going to eject first.

As our home life teetered between managed chaos and Hell, it was time for a visit from the two people I feared most—my mother and my doctor. It is downright shameful that the only thing I dreaded more than a doctor's visit was a check-in from my wonderful family. Yet both events shared similar qualities—concerned faces overshadowed by words of care, all of which made my heart heavier with every visit.

The doctor, however, was crowned as my number-one dreaded individual. And when he insisted I weigh in two days later, I found myself at a freight house, loading my mass onto a scale meant for cargo, not human tonnage.

"You are a brave man," a warehouse worker shouted to me. "Good luck."

Words of encouragement echoed as I shuffled through the packing-room to a truck scale. And like an 18-wheeler, I steered my mass to the platform's center. Red numbers flashed on the far wall; 550... 600... 650. I was 650 pounds!

Before that day, I could have only guessed my weight, but now there was no denying it, and with knowledge came gut-wrenching fear, not just of death but of change.

Will I have to give up pizza?

When I say I was worried about pizza, the average person asks, who picks death over a slice of pizza? Of course, no rational person would consciously choose addiction over life, but this is where my mind went, not to the outcome but rather the sacrifice.

Can I do it? Am I strong enough? The concern was not only for my eating habits and/or lack of exercise, but that I would have to face *what* made Dan eat. I had no idea what was under my rock of dysfunction.

What's the point anyway? I mulled over the problem later that night while sitting in a big-boy chair. *I've let my wife, my family, my friends, and even myself down. How can anyone forgive me when I cannot forgive myself?*

At 650 pounds, the pain is excruciating when attempting to get up from a seated position; muscles are weak, and joints hurt from inflammation. But I wanted to take a good look at myself, and no pain was going to stop me.

First, I maneuvered to the edge of the recliner, bracing a hand on the corner, and wobbled to my feet. As I shuffled down the hallway, my palms pressed out to the walls for balance until, eventually, I stood in front of the bathroom mirror. The room was dim, but I could see my splotched and bloated reflection—a visual reality I could no longer ignore.

You're a piece of shit. I could not think of anything worse to call myself.

My girth was braced on the side of the sink, and leaning forward, my stomach flopped into the porcelain basin. The edge dug into my skin, stinging, but I did not move. I could hear my heavy breathing, overwhelming an eerie quiet that filled the room. The bathtub dripped from behind me, a steady ping with a rhythmic pace I began to follow.

Ting. Ting. Ting.

Tommy must be asleep. My attention flickered to the quiet house. *Is Renee even home?*

Ting. Ting. Ting.

Why would God allow such misery in my life?

Get real

Ting. Ting. Ting.

God, yes. What about Him? Where is He? Beelzebub cleverly asked.

Sweat ran down my face, soaking my nightshirt. I glared at my reflection, considering Daniel Wayne Hawthorne, the walking, or rather, barely walking, face-of-death. I reflected on my family's recent visit and the pictures I posed for, like death on film.

You are already dead. There's photographic proof!

A wave of sadness washed over me. A shoulder-shaking, earth-quaking bucket of crocodile tears fell down my face. My body went limp. I was standing by the sheer law of physics, or maybe, sink fasteners made by Nasa. I laid my forehead to the steamy mirror, my cheeks slippery on the glass. Blood rushed my veins, injecting me with a warmth that had every limb on fire.

There is no going back. And a curious thought flourished; *life before today is flawed.*

I never considered myself a religious man; I was more of what some might call a spiritual person. And if I am honest, I was far from that man too, no longer able to see the beauty in life. I questioned God, debated his existence. If God were real, then why would a monster like me exist? I was a good guy. I was honest, never cheated or stole. So why would God let this happen to me?

I was angry at the Almighty for not taking the pain away. And yet, while leaning against the wall on that night in August, it was to Him that I prayed. As much as God angered me, He was my only hope. I screamed out, *Please. I will do anything. Just help me, God help me.*

***

A thunderous pounding shook the walls on what I now call the day after my mirror moment. "Dude, I gotta pee. Let me in."

My eyes flashed open, and I took note of my surroundings—the grey tile I sat on, a door bouncing at my back, my thick legs sprawled out in front of me.

"Give me a minute." My voice broke as Tommy pushed harder against my back.

When the door cracked, Tommy saw a 650-pound man sitting on the floor with his back against the only entrance.

"Oh shit, what happened?" He pushed, helping my girth with a forward motion towards the toilet, where I rested an elbow to the lid.

Upon entering, Tommy offered me a hand, and I glared at him. He was lucky to weigh 150 pounds, no match for my weight.

"Help me over there," I pointed to the edge of the tub, where I began to hurry my body, and the two of us pushed and pulled me to my feet.

"Please, help me to my chair," I quickly implored, cutting off the questions that were sure to come.

"What in the world happened?" Tommy watched in wide-eyed wonder as I flopped into my recliner, a sigh of relief exploding from my chest.

"I slipped."

Tommy did not do drama unless it involved him, and I knew how to distract him off the scene he had witnessed.

"Look, Renee doesn't need to know about this. I'll buy you a cold beer on Friday."

"I don't do beer, but you can buy me a bourbon and coke." Strutting back to the bathroom, Tommy chatted about where and when he could take me up on my offer, but I was not listening.

A miracle had happened—a visitation of truth, or a realization of life. A burden had lifted. And where I once feared change, I found myself contemplating it, mapping out a game plan; what should I do first, go to a gym?

What foods do I change?

It was as if someone had turned my internal key, and understanding resonated. My entire way of life was about to be altered. And I knew this to be true like I knew my eyes were brown and the sun rose in the morning. It felt natural. Up to this point, I had never stepped foot in a gym. I did not know the first thing about nutrition, but for the first time, I wanted more than the crumbs of life. I wanted the whole cake!

When I was 8, I felt like the man-of-steel, solid and unbeatable, but a time comes when everyone needs help. Batman needed Robin. The Lone Ranger needed Tonto. And I needed my family; it was that simple.

They don't know how to help you. Beelzebub was right. This was not my family's burden. It was mine.

But I could no longer hide from the truth; I had been a liar for years! I would say I ate salad when I had eaten a Big Mac. I would fib on my weight at the DMV, listing my 600 pounds as 350. The list of significant tales I have told over the years could fill the pages of this book. And while those white lies may not seem like much to some, I longed to feel good about my efforts towards a better life.

"Energy goes where energy flows," I had heard a television host tell his audience some months prior, and the thought had stayed with me.

The idea is that if we flood our lives with the positive and cut out the negative, the good light will overpower the dark corners. And at this point, negativity had been the master of my life. My dark spirit even had a name—and Beelzebub had had free reign for far too long.

With no plan formulated, I instinctively felt the first step was to banish negativity from my life. So I sat down with a pen, and on the back of an old envelope, I gave myself a reason for why I deserved a better life.

Why do I deserve to be healthy? Because I cared for others deeply. And now I permitted myself to care for me.

Why do I have the right to happiness? Because I was a giving person. What goes around comes around, and it was time for the spirit that I gave to shine on me.

Why do I deserve love? Because I loved easily.

Why should I be happy in a crowd? Because I was fun.

How is this going to work? I was patient. I'd figure it out.

That morning in August, I looked over the words I had written to paper, filled with an odd sense of accomplishment.

I am generally not a journaling man, but when I wrote, I felt free. *My change starts here*; I knew this to be true. I made a choice. Life over death. Love over rejection. Good over evil.

Chapter Six

Find Support

Angels do exist.
~ Journal entry 2010

Outside of broadcasting, I could not remember what made me happy. What were my goals, my ambitions? And at 45 years old, with half my life behind me and no real career, the path forward was unclear.

I was starting over. The idea frightened me. What was my purpose? Did I even have one? I was not in touch with my personal self. No one had ever asked me what I needed. And now, motivated by that night in August, I realized, I did not have to settle. I deserved to be happy. The change was up to me. Not my wife, not my family. No one else was responsible for my happiness. So, when a chance came to move back to Hagerstown, Maryland, I was ready to go home.

Find Support

Returning home required that I humble myself to my family. They knew only the story I had been telling them for the last 10 years—'Renee and I are fine, we are happy, and I am working on getting healthier.' Those were all lies. We had fallen apart years ago, I was dying, and I was broke.

When I left Hagerstown, I was headed to a dream radio gig at the beach, and I told all my friends and family I was going to be a big success. Now I was going back, and I would have to face these people as a very changed man. They were going to see me, hundreds of pounds heavier, no job, and walking with a cane. I was going home a total mess, but I made myself a promise to only move forward.

Do not look back; you're not going that way. I wrote the commonly heard statement on the next page of my makeshift journal. I needed a fresh start, and who else but family can give unconditional love?

"I really appreciate you helping us load up."

My big brother, Bill, had driven the three hours to Ocean City to offer his truck for the move home. And as he loaded his truck with our few belongings, my pride took an extra beating. Not because my big brother had come to my rescue, but because I was 650 pounds and practically immobile, so basically, I sat on the steps and watched. And Bill never once complained.

What will people say when they see you? Beelzebub lurked in the shadows, tossing my fears into the light of day.

I was 350 pounds heavier than when I left. I would have to deal with the dreaded looks from old friends and foes alike. *I must fight the urge to hide,* I knew. But I cringed over the thought, dreading its truth and the fear of judgment, which would only contribute to my negative dialog.

It's funny what the passing of a day can bring, because less than 24 hours later, I found myself sitting in a basic, one-bedroom apartment on the wrong side of the tracks in Hagerstown, Maryland. Everything was donated, from the couch and bed to the discounted rent, a gift from the state. Life was not grand, but it was affordable, and we were home.

What do I want from life? I wrote the question while sitting at an aluminum kitchen table, complete with red vinyl chairs and a single light overhead to highlight the big question.

I stared at the blank drafting pad, passing the time by sketching a caricature of Fred Flintstone in the margins. As always, he was grinning up at me, adorning caveman attire and hair like Elvis. And directly below E-Fred's necktie, I began my list…

1. Love, I want to feel loved.
2. Health, I want to walk, run, and bike through life.
3. Success, I want to make my mother proud.

Find Support

4. God, I want to make God happy.
5. Purpose, I want to discover why I am here.

As I looked over the list, I considered the simplistic nature of it, an average person's expectations of life. Doesn't everyone want some, if not all, these sentiments? And if the answer is yes, then how much is within our power and how much is pre-ordained? I pondered the idea, conjuring up a claim from childhood—declaring a grateful heart is where joy begins.

Skeptical and yet curious, I penned, 5 *things I'm grateful for*, at the top of yet another blank page. The pen toddled in my hand, hovering over an empty page, my mind searching for words.

"I must be doing this wrong," I sighed, my attention meandering to the smoke-stained walls and an overall smell like that of mold.

Should I be grateful for this? I considered the room, rethinking my new life in a neighborhood called Washington Gardens—aka the murder capital of Hagerstown. We had only been back a day, and already a drug bust had taken place, and a woman had stabbed her husband in the apartment next to us.

You came back for this? The negativity I hated echoed, and shaking my head, I turned another page, and this time wrote, F*ive things I am grateful for in Washington Gardens.* The pen was swift.

1. I'm not in Ocean City with Tommy.
2. I'm alive.

3. My family is here.
4. I am hopeful.
5. That husband stabbed last night was not me!

I pushed back from the kitchen table, eyeballing my words as if they might return a snappy retort. Beelzebub had impeccable timing, but no afterthought bantered back. Smiling, I crossed my arms and relaxed my shoulders, relishing in a foreign feeling of accomplishment.

"I will get healthy or die trying," I reaffirmed, and judging by the neighborhood, death by gunfire was a real possibility.

From that day forward, I rose early to escort Renee off to work, and then with a notepad and a phone book in hand, I would journal my 5 daily thanks before scanning for fitness advertisements in the local paper. At 650 pounds, the only exercise a man my size could safely participate had to be low impact, so swimming was an easy choice. And right there, under a list of local hotels, I saw "The Plaza Hotel Swim Club," for guests and residents alike to come and enjoy the pool, for a fee of $30.00 a month. We are all weightless in water; it was perfect. Easy on my body, good for my confidence, an obvious plus-plus, and from 7 AM until 10 PM, the pool was mine.

On that first morning, happy to find that I had the pool to myself, I jumped in on the 8-foot side. And because buoyancy is a gift to all overweight swimmers, I floated in place, treading water. When bored, I would

Find Support

switch it up, hang onto the sides and paddle like a mad man. Soon, I met other people, heavy souls needing friendship and inspiration. This was my first accurate understanding of how important others can be to one's recovery.

In the beginning, words of encouragement were very important. They helped me build a case, proving I was likable and worth it. Sure, if someone had rudely asked, "Why don't you go on a diet?" I would have forced out a joke and then later used chocolate to ease my pain. Though I worked to hold negativity at bay, I was not over my addictions or habits.

But the other dreamers at the pool kept me accountable. Watching them labor, fighting for their life as I did mine, allowed me to appreciate our similarities. And when I realized my family was rooting for me, well, I wanted to succeed even more. I longed to see my mother look upon her son with pride, rather than worry. I dreamt of the day when my sisters did not need a size update at every birthday or Christmas. I just wanted to feel 'normal,' whatever normal meant to me, my sense of it and not what the world labels me. And in the beginning, I admit, the desire to not disappoint those around me kept me from a candy bar. But hey, it was a start! And in time, I would learn how important it was to be good for Dan.

There was no real instructor, so I did my best to keep things positive at the new swimming hole. The movement was organic in nature. I encouraged those around me, easily giving away what life holds back from many—appreciation and acknowledgment. "You're a natural Donna," and, "Can you show me how you did that, Randy?"

The feeling of acceptance was contagious and nurturing. When people were done, they went out into their day sharing the experience. Soon, more folks came, everyone wanting a taste of what we were giving—hope and love. I was astounded to see how many folks were as unfamiliar with fitness as I. And what we learned from each other was shared, overall easing the anxiety about this new world of swim for everyone.

"Did you have to get a doctor's approval?" asked a man I recognized as Ted, a well-respected Hagerstown resident with connections to the Antietam Battlefield.

"No, I saw the advertisement," I said off-handedly while Ted treaded water next to me. "And I thought, why not?"

"Why not indeed?" we both agreed.

Ted was a big fella, funny, loved 50's music, especially Elvis. So it was for all those reasons we became swift swimming pals, passing the time discussing our relationship with food. As we paddled until exhausted, we discussed mutual struggles and fears. And though Ted was fifteen years my senior, he too measured life by the levels of pain and loneliness suffered. When he thought no one was looking, his attentions drifted faraway, as if he were reliving a lost dream. The resemblance between two lost souls compelled me, motivated me, casting a light on a purpose I would soon understand.

***

The winter of 2010 was bitter cold. So when my friends Doug and Cheri from Ocean City suggested we drive to Memphis for Elvis-fun and warmer weather, the four of us, including Renee, loaded my GMC and hit the road.

As it happened, Doug and I had connected over a mutual love of Elvis Presley. For the life of me, I cannot recount how many friends have come into my life because one man from Tupelo, Mississippi, took the world by storm in 1956. But Doug, a thin-faced slight of a man with a happy persona, shared a love for music I related to. He doted on his wife Cheri, opening doors for her, encircling her whenever she sat close. He seemed to always be touching her, feathering her blonde hair, and I wondered if after 20 years of marriage, whether it was automatic or intentional. Cheri stood at half her husband's height, and Doug called her his 'doll,' which always made her blush. Where Renee and I failed in the relationship department, Doug and Cheri were over achievers.

Doug had been given horrible news the month prior—he had cancer. And though his time on earth was to be short, a trip to Memphis held importance to Doug, and to me. For this was his last wish. So I drove and Doug sat shotgun while Cheri and Renee relaxed in the back. To this day, the 10 hours that Doug and I talked Elvis on the way to Memphis is a most cherished memory.

I told him how the last time I had gone to Memphis, I'd been in my 20s. And back then, I was much, much healthier, so this trip had me a bit nervous. First and foremost, I was afraid that I would not be able to enjoy the town like I had before. Outside of the pool, I had no stamina for moving around in the real world. Secondly, there was a huge Elvis fan club event taking place, and as a member of Elvis International, I was sure to meet people who, up until that point, had never seen me in person.

As most people do online, I hid my identity, often using younger or thinner photos of myself. Many members came from the United Kingdom, and while we had only chatted for a short time, I called them friends. While everyone was overly excited, I was deathly afraid of rejection.

We rolled into town late that next afternoon and the joke was on us, as Tennessee was under a winter storm warning. The Memphis area was colder than where we had come from, but we only laughed. Nothing could dampen my and Doug's excitement. We were in Memphis, which is like Disneyland to people who love Elvis.

Elvis music played everywhere we went, or I should say, everywhere I *attempted* to go, because I often lagged, allowing the others to go on ahead. My heart had a desire, but with temperatures below zero, my body would not move more than a few paces before every muscle cried out in pain.

We all took the tour of Elvis's beloved home, Graceland, but when I refused a wheelchair, I sealed my fate and saw little to nothing. Doing more sitting than touring, my focus was now on the pain rather than the tour. How I longed to return to that first visit in 1987, when a younger and happier Dan was up to his ole mischief, mimicking Elvis's voice in his own home.

I remember how my friend Jimmy and I stood in the front foyer of Graceland, while an older couple pushed for a closer look at Elvis's sitting room. "Do it, man. Do it," Jimmy encouraged with an elbow to my side.

"No," I hissed. But then he shot me a be-a-man look, the one all young people fall for, and so, I said in my best Elvis-like voice, "Man, I wish y'all would get the Hell out of my house."

The couple looked up, as if the voice came from heaven, while a young tour guide rolled a glare my way. Then, finally, the husband-and-wife team turned to see the big grin on my face.

"The big man did it, the big man, right there!"

The Giant in Me

Even in my twenties, I was thought of as a big man. *Now here I am, sitting on a bench 20 years later, unable to finish the tour.*

I cannot do this. I shook my head, watching as people passed with a familiar excitement on each face. *Next time, I will be a new man.* The promise staggered like a deflated balloon.

"Can I help you?" asked a man with Graceland Staff embroidered across the shoulder of a blue windbreaker. "Do you need a wheelchair?"

I should have said yes, but instead I heard myself utter, "No. Thank you. I'm working up the energy to walk back to the bus."

I pointed towards Meditation Garden, Elvis's final resting place and the pickup point on the far side, only to then realize the distance. My gut churned in anticipation of the pain. The man gave a sympathetic nod, then left me to work out how that might happen, and I imagined the trek to be slow and relentless.

As I trudged, each step heavier than before, I kept my eyes low. While fellow enthusiasts stood around Elvis' grave, I walked past, hoping to draw as little attention to the crossing giant as possible. While the sound of water trickled from a fountain nearby, emanating a sense of peace for all, I felt nothing.

"Are you coming?" Doug had broken away from his position near the grave to check on me and my curious exit.

Find Support

Paying our respects was something Doug and I had talked about the entire drive. It's ever Elvis fan's dream, to visit Graceland and leave a word of gratitude for a man who gave us a lifetime of music. But in this moment, I did not care.

"I'm not coming," I said, and the anger swelled alongside the physical pain. "I'll never come back here again, until I can walk through like a normal person."

I could feel Doug's sympathetic gaze at my back, as I shuffled to the bus. He was sad; I understood it. And while his disappointment was tangible, I was infuriated. I hated being the one that people pitied.

Oh, look at the poor guy trying to walk. That unfortunate soul, he's so fat, he's never going to make it. I imagined these exact words, and the more my mind lingered over this narrative, the faster my gate. Soon, I flopped my body to a bus seat and felt the van rock from a sudden shift. Happily, the driver was not onboard, so I sat and brooded alone.

Later, back in the hotel, while trying to decide which pair of gym pants did not look like sweatpants for evening wear, I contemplated my next step to kicking obesity to the curb.

The pool was a good start. *Check*, I made a mental note. And because I was not alone in my struggle, support was essential. *Check-check*.

I went to the lobby early, allowing Renee some privacy and alone time. As I entered, I was happy to see

Doug was already there. And I smiled, thankful when he returned a wave, showing no sign of uncomfortableness. What had happened earlier was gone. We were just two husbands waiting on their women and a night out on the town.

As Doug discussed the driving directions over a cup of hotel coffee, the question of where to find support consumed me. My mind fluttered from living in the moment to contemplating the future. And it was not until we were halfway to Elvis International's Dance Party that it dawned on me; I was about to see friends, face-to-face, for the first time! I could not hide behind an old photo. There was no GIF or silly meme to toss out when uncomfortable.

This meetup was happening! I cringed, glancing down to my tan moccasin slippers.

Yes, I was going to a party in sweatpants and carpet sliders. While others would flash their finest threads and fanciest shoes, I looked like a man settling in for a night of popcorn and movies.

I have truly reached the bottom.

As we entered the ball room, strobe lights bounced, while strangers were instantly inside my orbit. Thankfully, we were early enough to have the pick of tables, allowing me to sit far away from the action. And once placed, I would not get up, not even to go to the bathroom! So, naturally, all beverages would be limited, and Renee was long in the habit of dishing two food plates, mindful of perceptions where mine was concerned. These are the unfortunate tasks the families of the obese learn to protect us from public judgment.

People danced in packs under a disco light that spun at the center of the room. The groovy glimmer added an ambiance, a glow to the already timeless beat of "Suspicious Minds," which reverberated throughout the room. Even those on the sidelines could not help but sway with drinks in hand, evoked by music and memories.

I did not dance. Nor did I sway. I sat, counting the minutes for when friends from the United Kingdom would come, eager to meet Dan Hawthorne, and finally discover the real me.

"Dan?" I heard a woman I knew as Lynn say my name. "Are you Dan from Maryland?"

"That's right." I was slow to stand, and then, adding a swooping arm gesture, added an unwitting traction to the obvious. "That's me!"

If she was shocked by my size, she did not show it. And my comfort level improved as she hugged me.

"Lovely! Just brilliant to meet you. It is about time!" And with that, she was gone. So, I stood there, bewildered. Like I'd been kissed in the park by a stranger, only one thought prevailing—*that was pleasant.*

I've heard it said that Elvis fans are caring people, and on this day, they proved the sentiment right.

The Giant in Me

Whether it was the smiles or the random conversations as they passed my table, the takeaway impression was of a family-like bond. And I felt a sense of acceptance on that night, and I did not want it to end.

From my seat, I watched Lynn, sitting at a table of what I presumed were fans from the UK. They were joyful women, drinking spirits and exuberating a thrill for life that I envied. I took notice of the husbands lingering on the outside parameter, like a kind of masculine protective circle. Eventually, my gaze drifted to a single woman. Seated center table, she was seemingly involved in every conversation, eyes flitting about and responsive to many at once.

Blonde and fair, I placed her in her 40s. She was a natural beauty with glowing skin—a gift easily conjured by genetics, and not a product bottle. And judging by how the other women leaned in close to share in her conversation, she was respected. While I watched, puzzled by the mysterious nature of female interactions, it hit me; I was observing Patricia Garber, the author.

Months prior, I had witnessed Patricia's online interactions with other Elvis International members, but we had never been introduced. The members were fascinated by her storytelling; the idea of creating fiction inside Elvis's legacy was interesting, even to me. But it was her witty response that pulled me into the conversation, as I found her humor refreshing. I admired the way she communicated with an easy elegance, minus any hint of superiority. This led me to wonder whether the real Patricia was anything like her online persona, because mine surely was not.

Cat's out of the bag now, isn't it, fatty? I frowned, reminding myself to install a Beelzebub off-switch.

I did not meet Patricia that night; I merely watched from afar, quietly calculating the future. *I will introduce myself,* next time, I inwardly thought. And then the rebuttal, *In your dreams,* echoed, and I gave a sigh.

Life had a strange way of siding with Beelzebub. So it was no surprise, when the very next evening, I found myself sitting at a charity event, and lo and behold, in walked that same fair-haired author. I must have involuntarily sucked in a breath because Doug immediately turned my way.

"Are you alright, Dan?" He laid a hand on my shoulder, and I slowly nodded.

There were four women in her group, and when Patricia took a seat in front of me, a trail of feminine perfume wafted around me. The scent was mild yet memorable, like a snowfall in March.

"Is your club donating money?" I heard Renee ask on my right, "Why are we here?"

Though my attention was purposefully forward, I felt Doug and Cheri looking to me, as if wondering the same.

"I believe they are," I answered, quick like, not wanting to miss a word that flowed from the row ahead.

"Are you nervous?" asked the older woman sitting to Patricia's left.

Judging by the way she laid a hand to her knee, supportive and tender, I guessed her to be family. Mom, aunt, or sister? I leaned in, as if to shift position for comfort. *No, not sister,* I decided.

"I'm very proud of you." The woman said, stroking the back of Patricia's head, as if to straighten an invisible loose strain.

Definitely her mother. I agreed. Then, I began to muse over the irony of this woman's unescapable presence—first at the dance party and now here—and unwittingly, I gave an audible chuckle, which drew unwanted looks from my wife. But I merely shook my head, suggesting she should pay me no mind.

My mood elevated. All this eavesdropping was exciting and dangerous, it gave me a rush. Yet, if I'd had any sense, I would have been rattled, afraid to be noticed. We had shared in many group conversations online, and though I knew who she was, I was now cloaked under the ruse of nerves. Spotting a familiar face was the last thing on her mind.

"Patricia Garber, and the If I Can Dream fan club of Washington State." When the announcer called out the author, everyone in her group flinched, including myself.

Find Support

I watched as she collected a few things, stood, and walked to the stage. She was the picture of ease, like she'd done this very thing many times before. And I found myself wondering if she had, believing her to be more elegant than the night before, dressed down in a grey Elvis t-shirt pulled casually over a black skirt.

"Who's that?" Doug asked, obviously reacting to my interest.

"The author, Patricia Garber," I said, as if I'd read all her books and knew the details firsthand. Which, of course I had not, and did not.

"What author?" Renee was just now catching up.

"An Elvis author," I repeated.

"Aww, who cares," she stated in true Renee style.

And as a spokesperson for the event handed Patricia a microphone, I sat up a little straighter. In front of me, the woman I'd coined as her mother smiled with pride.

"I'm Patricia Garber," she began, and for three minutes she shared how the world of Elvis had embraced her stories, and in turn, she would like to donate her royalties for 2010 to Cerebral Palsy.

She went on to explain how CP had affected a member of her family, and the room clapped. A part of me filled with a sense of pride. Not in the same manner as I'd witnessed from her believed-to-be mother. But more like an acquaintance, who's living the moment with her, through association. I felt pleased to simply know her. Only, I did not.

At least, not yet.

CHAPTER SEVEN

BABY STEPS

*Broccoli isn't bad, but I'd rather have
ice cream.*
~ Journal entry, 2010

ONCE HOME IN MARYLAND, I QUICKLY settled into a new routine, less to-go foods and more prepared meals like chicken and fish. My understanding of good nutrition was limited, but I focused on eating more vegetables and drinking water.

Soon, I told myself, *I will be ready to weigh in, soon.*

I felt good about my food changes. My sweatpants required a tighter cinch; I was losing weight! Simple food changes and a swim schedule allowed for a noticeable loss of inches, loose shirt collars, and buttons that no longer strained against the fabric. But I was afraid of the scale, fearful it would remove the accomplishments that lifted my confidence.

My pants are loose, I wrote inside the pages of my daily journal. *This is finally happening!*

Each triumph sparked hope, and for the first time, success felt tangible. I was stronger, ready to move past the discomfort and the humiliation, looking to toss my emotional baggage aside and help myself.

That following day, high on achievement, I donned a new pair of checkered swim trunks and strutted to the pool. At the front door, I noticed a hung note: *Pool club will end on February 2nd, 2010.* I stared at it, defeat rushing like a deadly tsunami. My breath was quick, my chest tight. The pool and the friends, what was I to do without them? I was finally losing weight; now, where would I go?

In the days that followed, many wrote letters to the powers at the hotel, provoked by a desperate need, but nobody wrote back. The pool closed as scheduled and never reopened. Looking back, the closing was my first roadblock to success. And the irony was that my desire to lose the weight, finally strong, was now thwarted by outside forces and not self-destruction. I had lived through so many false starts that I stopped counting the failed efforts. However, I was now doing everything right, and yet, it was getting harder, not easier.

A light of hope came when an advertisement for a local gym caught my attention. The slogan suggested that no judgements were allowed through the doors. I had never walked through the front door of a gym and not felt as if I were a warning sign: *Attention, don't let this happen to you!*

Nervous, I went inside for a tour. Still using a cane, all eyes fell to me. Admittedly, I was a sight to see. I wore no gym shoes, only slip-on's because laces were impossible to reach. And while most of the equipment was foreign, the stationary bike looked familiar, so I tried it on for size and…did not fit. From then on, I eyeballed every piece of equipment with suspicion.

How do heavy people manage machines built for the fit? I was too wide, too large, to squeeze my girth onto most devices. *Except for a treadmill,* I considered, looking at one close by and imagining the 911 call.

"9-1-1, what's your emergency?"

"We have a 650-pound man down on our exercise machine!" Or, "We have tried lube, we have pulled and pushed, bring the jaws-of-life!"

This will not be pretty. As it was, I knew virtually nothing about cardio. I had to start somewhere, but I needed something elementary. What that was, I had no idea. Gutted, I turned to leave, pausing at the front desk and the young man working there.

"Excuse me, is there somebody I can speak with about getting help?"

The young man pointed to a lady at a table across the room. "She's our in-house trainer. Start there."

I approached the table, put my hand out, and said, "Hello, I'm Dan, and I really need help."

She was slow to look up from the clipboard, and when she did, eye contact was brief, as if looking at me was painful.

She took my extended hand and stated, "By the looks of things, you need to do at least six weeks of cardio before we can seriously work together. So sign the book, and I'll get back to you."

Her words hit me like a slap in the face, sharp and swift. Then, as she returned to her clipboard, I wondered why she did not see my potential. Was it not a trainer's dream to save a dying man and earn serious bragging rights?

Maybe I am not a challenge but rather a nightmare, I considered.

Then, I did not sign the book.

***

We are more vital than we realize. I believed this truth, yet I spent years abusing my body and spirit, forgetting that resolve is paramount.

Others cannot fix our problem; only we can. However, in my early stages of rediscovery, I struggled, much like a drowning man, lashing and reaching for anything, even if it was wrong. For a time, I gave reality weight loss TV a consideration, and even gastric bypass. Stuck in fight mode, I felt vulnerable.

I even went so far as to reach out to the producers of ABC's Extreme Weight Loss TV show, taping a humiliating audition video of myself, bare chested, as if parading my obesity around was completely normal. Horrified and desperate, I eagerly waited for them to email me back.

At this point, I only wanted the pain to stop. And if that meant I had to flash my girth for a few hundred million viewers, I was game. They promised to provide food and fitness instructors, which was greatly needed. I'd been stumbling down this health and wellness road, alone, for a few months, and I still did not understand basic nutrition.

An explosion of hope came when they answered back and offered me the job. I was finally going to get my life back! Someone wanted to help me!

For the next few months, I rode the waves of change like a rookie. I signed papers without proper representation, though they highly recommended it. I read over the travel requirements, as the show was to be taped in California, not considering the stress of being so far away from home during this time of change.

"Can you believe it, Renee?" I asked, flapping yet another paper in need of signing through the air. "This is really going to happen."

"How much will they pay?"

I stopped frolicking. "That hasn't been discussed," I said, trying to sound confident while my mind flashed through old emails. Had it *ever* been mentioned?

"So, it's not really set yet."

She has a point, idiot, Beelzebub chirped and I felt my chin drop.

30 days passed. And still, no word from Hollywood. I spent hundreds of hours hovering over my email, rereading old and writing new correspondences that were never sent. When the answer finally came, my fingers quaked as I moved the curser over the email and clicked to open. "We're sorry," was as far as I bothered to read.

The show had been canceled.

My soul plummeted into despair. I cried. I questioned. I screamed out into the night, the injustice of my life. Why was this so hard? Why would God not flip a switch and send me a little bit of luck? While I teetered on the brink of giving up, I lived inside a fog, everything muted and murky. Every day was the same, I would scan social media and the internet, my mind looking for answers my heart had already decided did not exist.

One day, a match was struck in my darkness. It was a soft light of hope, and it came by way of email, from a man who claimed to be Richard Simmons. To this day, I cannot remember if I had reached out to Richard in those days of confusion, but what I do remember were his words of hope. I must have told him about all my failed attempts, the pool, the TV show and the gym, because he responded with such grace.

"Rely on Dan Hawthorne," he said. "Make better choices, smaller portions, move your body as much as you can, and never give up."

This was my answer on the most simplistic level, and I could not believe Richard Simmons, the guru of fitness himself, gave me this excellent advice. He had taken the time to encourage me when nobody else had. It was unreal. I had been watching him help millions of people just like me, and now he was speaking to me.

The best part came at the end of his email, when he called me his "strong friend." To this day, we have never met. But if he is reading this—and I hope that he is—then he must know that he genuinely was a candle in my dark and scary room.

He said what I needed to hear: "Rely on Dan, my strong friend."

Meanwhile, unbeknownst to me, another angel was hard at work in my corner. Ann and I were high school friends who had not seen each other in more than twenty years. Our meetup was strictly by chance, but months later, she confided, "Every time we spoke, there was an underlining cry for help. And I just could not turn my back on you."

Ann's response to the vision of a friend in trouble was the turning point. For when she cared enough to send a single email, asking help for a friend, that young coworker Ann wrote to was Thomas Burge, the fitness director at Hagerstown Community College. And that friend in need was me.

One bright fall afternoon, I was summoned to Hagerstown Community College (HCC). I remember sitting in my car, warmed by the sunshine that streamed through the windshield, and yet frozen by fear. I sat there for over an hour, listening to my internal voice arguing with my apprehension.

Do not go inside. You will be a laughingstock! Beelzebub argued.

Meanwhile, the good chimed in for counter debate. *This is your chance to get real help. Isn't that what you want?*

A few weeks prior, I had spoken to Thomas over the phone, and in these short conversations, I discovered Thomas was new to HCC. And judging by the excitement I heard in his voice, it was apparent the fitness center was like a new baby. He wanted it to be a success. He explained to me that the gym was currently being used by the college faculty. The community did not know the facility existed. Both Ann and Thomas explained that by helping me, the word would get out, and the new gym would inspire the community—a win-win for all involved.

Timing is everything, and this was perfect. Over many phone conversations, it became clear that

Thomas knew of my struggle; he knew that I had been trying to get my life back and had faced disappointing developments along the way. And now, he wanted to talk face to face!

My nerves were up. I wanted Thomas to like me, help me, and, of course, not judge the book by its bloated cover.

The student parking was a hundred yards from the main entrance, and while I sat in my car, I eyeballed the path with trepidation. *That's quite a distance*, I moaned, praying I didn't hurt myself before arriving to the man's office!

As I walked down the first sloped path, my balance was off-kilter, and the pace was slow. It was maybe twenty steps before I got to the lower level, where I took a seat on a bench. From there, it was about fifty more steps to the front door, and I huffed and puffed as I walked the distance. My ankles and knees, as well as my back, were screaming.

Clearing the front door, I leaned on the wall next to the elevator and let my breath settle. Once up to Thomas' floor, I had to make another stop, as I did not want to enter his domain winded and sweaty. I am not sure why this mattered; it was not as if Thomas couldn't see the mess for himself, upfront and personal. But for my own self-pride, I wanted to walk in on my own two feet, upright and not dragging.

Thomas stood on the other side of the gym, lifting weights, but he quickly saw me and motioned for me to have a seat in the office to my right. A few minutes later, he came in, shut the door, and the journey began. I was sweating profusely while he asked questions. What had I tried before? What was I currently doing? He asked me about food; what was I eating? And I got the distinct feeling he was gauging whether or not I was mentally ready.

We talked about my food concerns, as it held a lead role in my life. I knew Thomas was not going to baby me. The fear of cutting out chocolate milk, which I had not yet done, was a real worry. Also, I was dreading the consequences of sugar withdrawals; what would that feel like?

Then there was Renee; how would I handle it when she wanted sweets? And she would not deny herself; she had made that clear. She was not the one looking to change. Could I handle her eating treats in front of me?

Up to this point, I had been making small changes, but I knew things were about to get tricky. I had no concept of food in moderation, and thought as most obese people do, that I had to give up all my favorite foods—forever! And for a person who feels food is everything, I braced for a level of grief, like that of a lost friend.

In the past, I concentrated so hard on what I could not have, until frustrated, I would give up. And to my relief, Thomas spent time explaining to me that, while I would initially be cut off from my favorite foods, it would not be forever.

"You will first need to control your intake while adding proper exercise," he explained. "Then, in time, we'll add some cheat days."

What was proper exercise? I wondered. And tell me more about those cheat days.

As Thomas spoke, the questions spun. What was common sense to most was a revelation to me. Basically, I thought skinny people ate everything they wanted while the rest lived in a constant state of self-discipline. And who could do that forever? Not me. So, the word "cheat day" was logged into my memory.

If Thomas were right, and I figured he was, a mix of moderation and reward might work for me. But, for my mental state, I needed awareness of a day to come, sometime in the not too far off future, when I could have anything I craved.

Food aside, my worry now turned to the fear that I would look like a clown in front of Thomas's gym staff. I had had enough humiliation. And I was not foolish; I knew people would be watching the 650-pound giant in the room.

The average person cannot resist watching an accident waiting to happen.

"We don't want to hurt you," Thomas explained. And then he added the words that started it all, "Go check with your doctor, and we'll get started."

The doctor's office was cold. And as I sat in the tiny, grey and white room, with a tangy scent of clean wafting around me, my stomach churned. I could hear voices outside my door, muttering female and male voices, all busy but none drawing close. Every fiber of my being screamed to leave, but I did not move. *I need the doctor's approval*, I understood. Or else Thomas could not help me.

"Good day, Mr. Hawthorne," the doctor began, eyes fixed on the chart in hand. "I hear you're wanting clearance to begin a fitness program?"

When his eyes finally looked up, I witnessed the same mental skip that plagues everyone when faced with the sight of a dying man. Quickly, he flipped another page, as if looking for the note he clearly missed, and then returned to me with a smile.

"Okay, well, good for you, Dan!"

I smiled and waited. There was more. When faced with this awkward dance, there was always more.

"At your last workup, you were borderline type two diabetes, and…" He flipped another page. "And, yeah, it looks like you've got some work ahead of you."

He said a mouthful.

"But, hey, let's get you up here on the table so I can listen to your heart."

Yes. The dreaded table, I thought, wondering if everyone hates this table as much as I do. The tiny step that no one's feet actual fit on but is necessary to hoist oneself up to the table of inconvenience. The paper cover that slides when you sit on it, thin, and bunching under my buttocks with every move. *Dreadful. Just awful.*

The best part of the whole ordeal? It didn't last long. And I walk out of there with a doctor's approval to begin working out.

And when my first day at the gym came, I was quieter than usual. I walked around, assessing my new environment, hearing the grunts and moans of people training around me. Thomas sat me down next to a hand-bike, requiring similar movements as a pedal bike only with one's arms, and asked me to do five minutes. I was happy to sit, as exertion while standing was brutal at my size. I was instantly sweating. And in fact, I had never sweated like that in my life, most certainly not by choice. Not even at the swimming pool, where if sweat was involved, I did not know it!

As Thomas moved me through a series of exercises, like the medicine ball toss to lat pulldowns, and some light dumbbell presses, I was quiet as a mouse. There was no way I was going to growl like some animal and draw more attention my way. Outwardly, I was mute.

While inside, I refuted the pain, reminding myself that I was doing this to save my life. And if I did not partake, I would eventually die.

When the first workout was behind me, I was still standing. Winded and hot, my confidence pumped with the achievement. It felt good to know that Thomas believed in me, or else he would not have asked me to come. The hurt was good, and with every step back to my car, my body reminded me that I had accomplished a remarkable feat!

I made it through the first day. I was revitalized.

Chapter Eight

The plan

My dinner plate is colorful, full of green and red; I've never seen anything like it.
~ Journal entry, 2011

I cannot lie; my old friend (food) was still on my mind. I would pass a burger joint on my way home and fight the urge to indulge. As much as eating healthy lifted my energy, some days, a greasy burger after a workout sounded like heaven. And my desire to satisfy became the new battle, and Beelzebub cheered me on.

Nobody is looking, an internal voice would say. *You can have a burger and a shake, you worked hard. You deserve it.*

And he was right. No one was looking. I could sneak a burger and shake. I would only be letting myself down. But I had just begun to feel the difference of a healthy routine, and I did not want to void the effort.

The Plan

I can wait, I counterargued. *I want to see results before the reward.*

In those first few months, I was successful 90% of the time. But on a few occasions, I gave into that burger and shake. The following day, I journaled the event and then reported the slip to Thomas.

"I have a confession, boss," I approached the subject gently.

"Yeah, what's that?" Thomas was seated at his desk, focused on a stack of papers.

"I had a cheeseburger after our workout yesterday." *There, I said it,* I thought, and a weight instantly lifted.

Thomas looked up, his face deadpan. "At a drive-thru or at home?"

Unsure where this was going, I hesitantly admitted, "A drive-thru," and then wanted to take it back when his face plunged in disappointment.

"A drive-thru? Dan, if you're going to cheat, cheat wisely. Make the burger fresh at home!"

My face must have been a picture of regret because he quickly added. "Look, today is a chance for better choices."

He really is the voice of reason. I smiled as Thomas went on to explain that accountability is necessary, that every day is a choice, and tomorrow, a new start. The goal is to stack one successful day after another, all the way to the finish line.

My sight was set on 300 pounds. And the first big shock came at the scale when even after many slips, I charted a 50-pound loss. Now at 600 pounds, I understood that even if I stumbled 10% of the time, success could not be stopped unless by me.

The idea that the human body is a fine-tuned engine when it's worked and fed properly was new to me. And from then on, I worked hard all week, and if the temptations crept up on me come Saturday, I would make myself a fresh grilled burger or chicken, light on the condiments, and big on onions and lettuce. For the first time ever, I was in control, not food.

It was good to be king.

Each new day started with a plan. The proposal began where the journey started, in front of the bathroom mirror, with daily goals and reminders that there will be no fast food on the run. And once I was out for the day, temptations would be addressed as they came. While I did not go looking for speed bumps, I was aware they existed, as denial only leads to failure.

It is better to face it and remember that while those foods may taste good, nothing feels as good as breathing and walking.

Nothing feels as good as being healthy.

We live in a fast-paced world where everybody wants something yesterday. That way of thinking was not meant for my weight loss journey, where goals needed to be realistic and straightforward. Staying with the

The Plan

positivity I had cultivated thus far, I sat down and wrote out what the workouts would be each week, based on Thomas's input, as well as the meals.

Advanced food preparation, Thomas drilled, and I learned it well!

My helpful tool—cooking up what was needed for the week left no room for a rushed choice under the pressure of hunger. The grilled chicken was always in my fridge, decreasing the opportunity for procrastination. The more ready, the better I did. And keeping with my routine made roadblocks easier to spot, and adjustments were quickly made. Hiccups of error were nothing more than a chance to stay in a positive forward motion.

"Hey, boss, how much can I lose each week?"

Thomas was clocking my circuit rotation, elevated pushups to hand ropes, following sit-ups—a CrossFit technic that he loved, and I dreaded.

"Time," he said, ignoring the question. Then a second later, "Go!"

This fast-paced routine took my breath, delaying my pursuit of the topic.

"Dan, it's too early for you to worry about that," he finally said while I grunted at his feet, "but if you lose one to three pounds a week, I'd say that's a safe goal."

All I needed to hear was a long-term goal of 8 to 10 pounds a month. And I used the same thinking as I did with food. If I can accomplish this goal 90% of the time, I should see victory. But if the scale is not kind, I told myself, I will focus on the next week, remaining realistic and patient.

Working with someone like Thomas was a game-changer for me. He helped with everything from food to adjusting my routine when the scale decelerated. I learned about healthy eating plans like Paleo, where everything is bought fresh, no box or bagged items, a farmer's dream. Thomas often switched workout routines, say, from a stationary bike to the treadmill or worked different muscles in order to boost my metabolism. Life at the gym was a constant challenge, completing me in a mind, body, and spirit kind of way that I had never experienced.

***

Meanwhile, on the home front, my routine was much like a job. I would wake at 5 AM, hit the coffee pot for two cups of Joe, and consume two eggs over-easy and a piece of whole-wheat toast with my first glass of water. Renee and I were off by 6 AM, and after dropping her off, I headed to the gym with a banana in hand.

When I first started, workouts were no more than 15 minutes. And once done, I would eat that banana with some cashews or almonds, all the while visiting and encouraging others working hard on their own goals. Once home, I was ready for lunch, which consisted of a big salad full of romaine lettuce, spinach, onions, chicken, and sometimes a bit of cheese. And on a similar day, like all the days before, the house was quiet while I folded the laundry, anticipating my 5 PM cue to pick up Renee.

One Tuesday, I parked behind Renee's place of employment and waited, flipping the radio dial while plotting a return to broadcasting. Time went by, but no Renee. At first, I told myself the boss must have delayed her, but I knew something was wrong when a full hour went by. So I went in, and after speaking with a coworker, learned that Renee had left earlier in the day.

She had left without a word.

Not even with all our dysfunction could I have guessed this would happen. And 24 hours later, after discovering that money had been withdrawn by Renee at an ATM in Tucson, I knew she would not be back. My mind struggled with my heart. On the one hand, I knew Renee could leap without a thought to the outcome. And it was likely that she believed she was on an adventure. But, on the other hand, I feared for her safety.

Let her go, my mind reeled. *She did what should have been done years ago. Let her be.* But what if she'd misjudged the company she kept? What if they were dangerous? *She knows nobody in Arizona!*

As the day slid on, I made more phone calls, questioning Renee's friends until I had an address. I needed to know that she was okay, that this is what she wanted. And I deserved, at the very least, to hear it from her personally. And because Tucson was a good 30-hour drive, I mustered up a friend.

Dale and I drove day and night alternating the wheel, and by late morning on the second day, we crossed the Texas state line. Finally reaching the halfway point, the car's air conditioning conked out, leaving us to drive the last remaining hours in face-melting Hellfire. And when we finally pulled into the address, we were a sticky, stinking hot mess.

The home was lovely, stucco style, typical for Arizona, and much nicer than anything Renee and I could have ever afforded. I knocked on the door, running a hand down my sweat-stained shirt. I remember thinking how I would not answer if I saw the likes of me standing on the other side. But a grey-haired lady did answer, looking quite perplexed.

"Can I help you?"

I explained that I was Renee's husband and asked to talk to her. "If that's okay with you, ma'am," I added.

The poor lady looked like someone had spit in her face, bewildered and affronted. "I wasn't aware Renee was married."

"I assure you, there will be no trouble." I held up my hands in a surrendering manner. "I just want to speak to her."

The Plan

"My son is at work," the woman said, looking me up and down as if deciding her next move. Then she closed the door, and a moment later, Renee came outside. She looked uncomfortable in her own skin, disheveled, but with no sign of harm.

"Are you okay?" I asked as Renee's eyes roamed around like she was only now realizing her surroundings. "Do you want to go home?"

Her fish-out-of-water appearance seemed like answer enough, but I waited.

"Yeah," was all she said, before turning to go inside to fetch her things.

The drive back to Maryland was long and mostly silent. Only Dale and I spoke, but daggers could be felt from the back seat. It was unclear who Renee was upset with more, me or herself, but I felt sure it was embarrassment that fueled her unspoken rage.

Once home, Renee stayed even more to herself. And when she did not ask me for a divorce, I resigned that I would end the nonsense. One night, while I sat on the front porch, rocking and watching the neighborhood, I plotted the future.

Renee could stay here, I thought. *I will move.*

I focused on what a separation would require from the porch while monitoring the Methodist church up the corner. It was hard to miss the chapel. People were constantly entering and leaving, families dressed smartly, smiling, and walking hand in hand. I longed for the peace that emanated around them, like a mist of happiness. I imagined joy, a rainbow inside the group, all while I was watching and working on my situation.

Why did Renee come back? The question kept circling, along with, *Did she feel sorry for me?* Of course, I imagined; anyone would find it difficult to leave a man who once could not walk.

But those days were over; I was slowly approaching a 100-pound loss. Finally, in the spring of 2011, the weight was melting off, and I was a happier man with a hopeful future. And though Renee did see my success, she only resented me more — a case of too little too late. So, while the end was filled with so many questions, a need to seek higher advice nagged at me.

Pastor Rick had a big smile and an even more welcoming hug. He did not know me from Adam — no pun intended — but after a quick inquiry, he invited me to a church fundraiser dinner that weekend. Nervous and excited, I wanted to get close to this loving spirit I had seen from afar, centering on the First Methodist Church in Hagerstown, Maryland. My clothes now hung on me like a potato sack, but I donned an Elvis t-shirt and went happily to what was essentially an indoor picnic.

Whenever Elvis is displayed, friendships spark. "Are you a big Elvis fan?" a lady with a captivating smile and a child attached to her leg asked.

The plan

"I am," I offered, already feeling welcome.

"Pastor Rick is going to want to meet you," she all but squealed. And thus began my relationship with the honorable small-town protector of souls.

Rick's embrace was big and firm, seemingly engulfing me, though I was much larger than he. His sincere greeting gave way to immediate trust on my part, but I did not want to ambush him with all my problems, so I took my time. And over the next few weeks, I went to Sunday service, joined in the worship, and made it a point to stop on the way out for the customary small talk.

This was so much more relaxed than the church I was raised in, where people became overcome by the spirit and spoke in tongues. At the age of 8, baffled by these oddities, I would mimic what I had witnessed, much to Nan's shock.

"Ah-be-da-duda-buta." I would toss back my head, hoping to accomplish an inward eye-roll because white eyeballs would be so cool!

"Daniel Wayne!" Nan yelled from the front seat, her belly jiggling with a need to laugh while the rest of the bus looked less amused. I may have only been 8, but I had it down like POW-Batman!

After a while, I became a familiar face at the Hagerstown Methodist Church and Pastor Rick knew my name on sight. There was always laughter as I exited the church, and a few times, we talked about gathering to enjoy Elvis music together, someday.

"Dan, I'd love for you to come and share your story with our congregation." The pastor held firm to our handshake. "And I even promise to play some Elvis afterwards, if you like."

We both laughed. "I would love that, sir," I said, and he waited, as if expecting more.

An awkward pause pulsated. And a pretext formed on my tongue as the eyes of eager patrons burned at my back.

"I've got to clean up a few things, in my life," I began, my gaze falling to the ground. "But once I do, we'll talk about doing just that. I would be honored."

As a recovering food addict, and the second party to a codependent marriage, I wasn't ready. My life at that point left me feeling unworthy of the task.

"Well, you let me know if I can help."

Help? Adrenaline heated my veins. *Of course, he can help!*

"I will do that, sir," I said, taking a quick step forward, only to spin back, grinning and pointing to the man of God. "You'll see, I am going to call you."

Chapter Nine

Expect Bumps

I'm in the driver's seat now, and food is the passenger.
~**Journal entry, 2011**

That old cliché "life is a challenge" rang true for most of my life. But now, the cards felt stacked, as temptation burned with the cutting pain of withdrawal.

Oh, look, it's Easter. Everyone is enjoying egg-shaped peanut butter cups, but you! Summer's here. Krumpie's donut shop will be open late, but not for you!

I would have laughed if someone had told me that to beat obesity, my daily attire must include a suit of armor. I should expect a fight, as there would be days when simple life forces are against me. Like how on a cold winter day, snuggled up in bed and dreaming nicely, the idea of a gym would turn my stomach. Or how, in the wee hours of the morning, I would awake to the whispering evils of sloth and gluttony.

You don't really want to go sweat like a drunken sailor? Beelzebub would taunt while I lay awake in bed. *You can catch up tomorrow.*

Battle fatigue is accurate, and it sinks in deep. My body reeled from the effects of a previous day's workout, my heart heavy, and my soul unwilling to take on another trying task. Nobody really likes pain and discomfort. Nothing comes easy on a journey to better oneself. If it were easy, we would all look like movie stars. And the physical battle, though small compared to my emotional challenges, was a tough challenge at the age of 47.

To combat disappointment, I journaled, filling page after page with my mental bile. And when journaling felt stale, I found myself writing poems, purging emotions to paper with a rhythm that I was unaware of. "A Man in the Mirror," by Daniel Wayne Hawthorne...

Who was that man in the mirror
looking back at me that night?
He was scared and lonely.
He was losing his life.

The mind and spirit had grown dark.
Wake up, wake up.
You're falling apart.

The Giant in Me

The will and desire were found from within,
but there were no tools.
Where do I begin?

Obstacles and challenges were there from the start.
But the desire to succeed flowed from the heart.

Win the battle; there must be a way.
You have so much to live for.
You have so much to say.

The problems got tougher,
Things were a mess.
Never give up.
Life is always a test.

Negativity was winning,
but out there was still hope.
Then an angel delivered
me a message in a note.

I want to help you. Are you ready to fight?
You have what it takes to get back your life.

The journey started; we formed a team.
We've come real far,
much more than I dreamed.

EXPECT BUMPS

There are many others in the mirror.
They're lost and feel trapped.
Part of this journey
is to always give back.

Inspire with your story.
Be a light.
Help them get started
to get back their life.

The man in the mirror, he found his way.
We all have a purpose,
and should appreciate every day.

Of all revelations, the idea that my story was not unusual was the one thing that changed my purpose. I had once believed my Hell was special, like the torture was custom built. The idea kept me hopeless, separated from the rest of the world, where many are suffering, but I had not been listening.

But that changed one unexpected day, when on my way to the gym, my car broke down. And because the walk was a good 10 miles, I located a city bus map and plotted my next move. According to the schedule, I could catch a bus up the street from where the car died, take it to Hagerstown City Park, where I would make a switch, and ride another bus the rest of the way to the college!

Perfect, I thought, and off I went, challenge accepted.

It was a rainy day, and for some reason, the bus arrived a few minutes late, but I got on, happy to finally be on my way. With stops included, it took about 20 minutes to get to the park, where my other bus was supposed to be waiting, but it was gone. I had missed it. But a friendly bus rider told me that another would be around in 30 minutes, so, I flopped down on a bench and focused on the good and not the day's bad luck.

At least the rain stopped, I mused, bracing for Beelzebub, who rarely missed a chance at a retort, but nothing came.

While waiting, a man sat next to me, close enough for conversation, and I instantly shifted away from the intrusion. Though I normally enjoy a chat with a stranger, on that day, I found myself calculating the odds of him choosing this exact seat, what with all the empty benches available. And from the corner of my eye, I peeked at him, noticing that he had only one hand, and then felt guilty for wishing he had sat elsewhere.

What had fate dealt this man? I wondered, while also calculating his age. *No older than 25,* I thought, as he suddenly blurted out, "I know you!"

I froze, eyes straight ahead.

"Aren't you that man that's losing all the weight?"

Politeness dictated I confirm I was indeed him, but something else seemingly guided me to explain further. I could hear my happy explanation of how the local newspaper was kind enough to publish an article, highlighting the college gym that was helping my new life. And though I was speaking, I felt as if I was hearing the story for the first time.

"I would like to thank you!" He offered me a handless arm.

I hesitated, hoping he missed the blunder, then took his wrist and gave a firm shake.

"I lost my hand while on a drug binge," he answered, like he knew my next question. "I passed out with my hand in the campfire, and it burnt right off."

The pain, the anguish, the idea left me breathless. "I'm so sorry to hear that, friend."

"Thank you, but I didn't feel anything. I was high." The young man waved it off. "I'm clean now, and I'm going to stay clean, and I want to thank you."

"Me? I'm sorry, I don't follow."

"I read your story, about how food is your addiction, like drugs are mine? And when I saw the before photos, man, you looked bad. So I figured if this guy could fight for his life, then I had to try."

"That's beautiful." The sentiment of community, of being connected to another living soul, filled the rims of my eyes.

"I've done a lot of bad things, stolen from the people I love, but you said we all have a purpose. Do you really believe that?"

"Yes! Absolutely! And it is just a matter of doing what's right, then giving back so another can discover their purpose too."

"I believe you, I do."

"Believe in yourself, friend. Tell that man in the mirror every day that he is beautiful, that he is worth it, and he deserves to live a happy, healthy, and clean life."

We were both misty, each lost in a life-altering moment we would never forget.

The young man hugged me before he boarded a bus to an unknown destination, and I stood in the cold, warmed by the experience. My thoughts kept circling, from the car that had broken down that morning, which ultimately led me here, to this young man. My heart was whole, re-sparking a conviction to help others as much as myself. Later, when the next bus arrived, I took it, damp but never more ready for a workout.

When I arrived, I walked down the long hallway, and young men and women passed, giving me high-fives with, "Good going, Dan. Keep up the good work," and youthful expressions like, "You got this, dude," pounding my fist to their own.

People genuinely care, the sentiment swelled. *The entire campus is on my side.*

For many months, I had noticed a shift at the college, where at first the campus staff and teachers were the ones that came, now more student-faculty were present for my early morning workouts. In addition, members of the track team came to meet, encourage, and workout with the man from the paper. The college felt like family, my home away from home.

Friends and strangers alike were invested in my journey, and I began to realize it was not just about weight loss. It was about the battle. Everybody loves a good fight; no one is immune from life's scars, but we love to see the underdog rise from the ashes to win. We all want the story to end with the good guy or gal on top.

When it was time for me to head home, tired from the day's challenges, I dreaded the bus ride. I could have called a taxi or even a family member, but I kept remembering my new friend and the experience that moved me.

What if there is more to learn from this day? I pondered as I walked to the bus stop, leaning into the wind.

With a few minutes to spare before the bus arrived, I sat down and took out my notepad, rereading words I had written earlier. *Anything can happen.* The sentiment filled me as a man walked up and sat one bench across from me. The hairs stood up on the back of my neck.

He was a young African American college student and, judging by the stack of books in his hands, a dedicated one indeed. He watched me in careful glances, discreet and yet forward, like he had something to say but questioned his motives.

"Do you mind if I sit by you?" The question conjured a warm, understanding grin, and I could not help but smirk in anticipation of the next miracle.

"Absolutely." I signaled to the open spot. "I'm Dan."

"I know," he said. "I saw you in the paper! Your story really helped me."

"Did it?" I turned to face him, searching his eyes for more blessings to an already fantastic day.

"I've been back to school for a few months, but the stress has been weighing on me, tempting me back to my old ways, the ways that landed me in prison."

"Prison is not where you belong," I automatically said, no backstory needed. "You must have dreams, or you wouldn't be here."

"I have many dreams." He was looking at the ground now. "And I want to thank you for sharing your story because before I read it, I honestly thought I wasn't going to make it through another day."

"Thank you for sharing that with me. It means a lot."

"You should think about lecturing. What you have to say can help many people like me."

Of course, I missed the next bus. I stayed to listen to the young man's entire journey, from his troubled childhood to his struggle in school and life on the streets.

"You know, the key is to love yourself enough to make it happen."

Before that day, I had never shared my love-you-first theory with anyone, and already I had shared it twice with two young men in one day. And both times, they flashed me a grin of skepticism.

"We have to love ourselves enough to make the necessary and often harsh changes."

He pondered that a moment and then gave me a nod that suggested he approved.

"The desire to change, or the knowledge that we need to, is not always enough." I continued to build my case, explaining how it's as if we have been charged with recklessness and now must evoke our right to life.

While we were speaking, a realization dawned; by helping these young men, I had discovered the point of my entire struggle. All the times I had questioned, why me? Why am I forced to suffer? Now I had my answer; in suffering, I can now help another. Through my struggle comes compassion.

When the young man boarded his bus for home, I looked up to the sky to an invisible God and shouted, "You're the boss! Whatever you say, I will do."

CHAPTER TEN

FIND YOUR INNER STRENGTH

I'm not always Superman. Some days I settle for being Robin, the boy wonder and sidekick.
~ Journal entry, 2011

ADDICTED TO TV BY CHOICE, I saw the weight loss commercials and heard all the variations of overnight success. It sounded easy. The promoter suggested that all one needs is to take a pill, drink a shake, or get with the latest fad.

But what if that mold doesn't fit?

The pitch attempts to remind us of the self-confident flair we once had. What's that, you ask, you have never been self-assured? You have been heavy your entire life? No worries, this magic elixir will fix that too!

False. All lies.

Willpower is something I knew little about; I denied myself nothing and instead cultivated a 47-year relationship with food. No pill could change my history. No stranger could teach me to dig deep. I had to turn my internal key on my own.

When I was 650 pounds, I considered many fix-it-quick regimes. I needed the fairytale to be authentic. And while the weight loss industry profits by giving hope to the hopeless, the core problem, like why we indulge, goes undiscovered. Though, out of desperation, I contemplated these alternate methods, I instinctively believed I needed more. Understanding why I overindulged was as necessary as an easy-to-follow routine.

Did I get enough sleep? Was I remaining positive, grateful, and mentally balanced? Did I eat a healthy breakfast before the gym? If anything was off-kilter, I could not expect to be lifting a 75-pound dumbbell or walking 5 miles on a treadmill. And as for willpower, that was out the window. I was weak to my urges.

In the early days, I gave no thought to the power of the mind, body, and spirit, nor how all three contributed to the success. If my head was not in the game, those 75-pound dumbbells suddenly felt like 150 pounds. And every mile walked was more demanding than the one before, which plunged my confidence.

Cultivating my inner strength became a daily routine consisting of faith, self-care, meditation, and proper nutrition. Every change made was a conscious decision, like cutting out the negativity from my life, both situational and relational. Although there was no magic pill to do the work, I did it, and the road was hard. My fears were many, and even once conquered, a new one would take its place.

After so many years of neglect, my body and I had to get reacquainted. And when I stayed true to the routine, I felt like Superman. But if I did not, my strength would wither, and the cause-and-effect outcome was quickly understood. However, the mind was another matter; for even my confidence had limits. I was slow to trust my body's capabilities, no matter sleep or food. After all, I was once a 650-pound man who struggled to reach the bathroom just a year prior. Hundreds of pounds gone, and still, I was slow to believe what my new body could accomplish.

Everything was a process, and the building up of my confidence was as important as understanding my body's inner system. I remember one day, about a month in, I decided to try bar squats. This is where a straight bar, stacked with weights, rests on one's shoulders. And when ready, one drops into a sitting position and then up again. Because my balance was not good,

FIND YOUR INNER STRENGTH

I asked Thomas and a friend to stand behind me, offering hands-on support.

For weeks, I had been watching others manage this exercise, and my heart was ready to try. But I honestly did not know if my body could handle the challenge. Obesity had distorted my ankle bones, and my knees were not much better. So, when I stepped under the bar, pressing my shoulders against the steel, my grip went sweaty and my arms quaked.

"I am having second thoughts." I blurted out, suddenly petrified.

What if my legs couldn't hold me, or worse, fell to injury?

"No, you're doing this," Thomas barked, stepping closer to me from behind.

My legs wobbled like months of training had never happened.

I don't care how much you've lost, you will always be a 650-pound giant! Beelzebub taunted, and I pushed the voice from my mind.

"This is a bad idea, boss," I could hear my voice pleading.

"Dan, you are strong enough to do this," Thomas said in my ear. "And we're staying here until you do at least one squat."

Thomas felt I could do this, I considered, trying to remember a time when he had been wrong. "Okay, let's try."

The Giant in Me

I lowered into position, the weight catching me by surprise, sending my legs muscles into involuntary quivers. I barely bent my throbbing knee joints before popping back up.

"You got this, Dan, trust me." Thomas patted my shoulder. "Try again, lower this time."

After another deep breath, I closed my eyes and finally dropped down, allowing my body a moment to adjust to this new world before attempting my first legal bar squat. I felt strength inside the pain, as if my tired muscles relished in the task, reminding me that the pain was from the effort, and not a premonition of failure. And once the squat was completed, I merely stared at my reflection in the mirror that faced me. What had just happened? Had I dug deep and suddenly tapped into a well of hidden courage?

Honestly, a process for success had been in place for months. First, I had a good night's rest, then woke and had a great breakfast. Second, I had spent hundreds of hours cultivating confidence and mental readiness in Thomas, as well as myself! Third, I had been at that gym every day, five days a week, strengthening my body for a prepared level of performance. And with all that done, I still had my mind to overcome self-placed obstacles from years of self-inflicted abuse. And even after all that, it still took two good buddies, standing behind me, encouraging me to try!

When all was said and done, I could not "just do it."

All anyone can do is ride that stationary bike or walk that treadmill for as long as one safely can. And if that is managed for only a few minutes, then the effort should be celebrated. The fact that I got up that morning, put healthy fuel in my body, and went to the gym counted for something. The fact that I did not spend the day on the couch watching TV was an accomplishment!

The world may try to tell us differently, but they have not lived our life. The emotional struggle of obesity cultivates deeply-rooted scars, often contributing to a more severe disorder that we cannot conquer alone. Our body and spirit need time to heal, and above all, we need to try!

***

After spring break, Thomas had begun to teach a health and wellness class at HCC, to which I was asked to speak about my journey. Of course, I owed Thomas everything—literally my life—so I was happy to help.

Many of the staff joined me for early morning workouts before classes started, and word got around that I would be addressing Thomas's students.

"Now, don't be nervous, just tell them exactly how you feel," Robert said.

Robert was in his early 60s and amazingly fit. He coached tennis and volunteered at the college gym during the week. He was much taller than me, and we were the two oldest gents in the room, so we bonded quickly. Robert was a genuine product of the free-loving '60s, accepting of everyone and everything.

His stories intrigued me. Like the time he had seen Elvis in concert, Baltimore, Maryland, in 1971. He was a diehard Beatles fan, he explained, and had gone to the Elvis concert out of curiosity. After all, how does one man, who the world calls the King, entertain the masses? Surely, there would be performed miracles, acrobats, and fireworks. But to Robert's surprise, the show was simple and yet mythical—one caped man and his band. And from that point forward, he was a fan, which made Robert golden in my book!

"You have done an amazing job," Robert said. "And after that tough first day, we were taking bets as to whether you would come back!"

"Did you? I chuckled. "I'm sure I was a scary sight."

"Well, in case you're wondering, I said you'd be back," Robert spoke in a hushed tone, leading me to believe some had an alternate view.

"And I did come back." I grinned.

On that Friday afternoon, in 2011, Robert wished me luck, and off I went to Thomas's waiting students. Finally, the guy who had struggled to graduate 12th grade had something to share with a college class. Who would have thought?

When I got to Thomas's classroom, my nerves were rattling. And I hesitated in the open doorway, expecting to see a room full of young people counting the minutes to the upcoming weekend. But instead, everyone was seated, eyes forward and attentive. My palms began to sweat, dampening the notepaper in my hand. And I cleared my throat, interrupting Thomas where he stood, his back to the class and writing something on a chalkboard. When he turned, he smiled, and I thought I saw a reflection of my own nerves inside his grin.

I had no fancy PowerPoint program, no colorful visuals, just a story fresh in my head. And as the hour passed, I told my story as bluntly and clearly as I could manage, making sure to reflect equally on the highs and lows. And in the end, I gave the floor over to the curious.

"Did you have trouble bathing at 650 pounds?" one young man asked.

"No. The myth of heavy people being dirty is false. We have no trouble showering."

"What about sex?"

The question admittedly shocked me, but I quickly retorted, "Do you mean with myself or with others?" And the room roared with laughter.

When my time was up, many students thanked me for the laughs and honesty. So, of course, I return the gratitude, appreciating the opportunity to spend an afternoon with such vivacious young souls. Though most of the students did not outwardly appear in need of my story, I did notice a young woman seated in the back.

She sat at a single table, with other empty desks strategically placed around her, like a fort to ward off the enemy. I thought her pretty, with fair complexion and auburn-colored hair. However, judging by her stand-off demeanor, she appeared unapproachable. After class, while everyone filed out, she lingered, allowing her classmates to leave before approaching me.

"I can relate to what you said." Her voice was slight, and as she spoke, she drew the books in her arms closer, like a shield of armor. "Can I ask you a question?"

"Yes, absolutely." I waved her closer.

"How do you deal with your bad feelings?"

This is a good question, I thought, one that I had hoped to be asked.

"I'm not going to lie, that's a tough one. But what helps is still the mirror. I look at Dan every morning, and I tell him he can do it. I tell him that he's important. I know this sounds a bit silly, but it does help."

She was smiling, eyes cast downward to her shoes, her body gently swaying for comfort while giving my words some thought.

"You know, journaling helps too. I find that purging all my bad thoughts to paper is a relief. And you can toss it in the trash later, which feels great."

That seemed to resonate, and she gave a light laugh.

"I just can't seem to get the food right. I like food too much, I guess."

"And we won't always get it right. I make mistakes occasionally too." I covered my mouth as if to hide the subsequent admission. "Like milkshakes and cheeseburgers."

We both laughed. It was good to see the young woman smile.

"Don't be too hard on yourself. It will be okay, and I'm in your corner."

When I left the campus that day, I was pumped and yet worried. I contemplated the talk; guiding a lecture was new to me and whether I had said enough or maybe too much was a concern. But my spirit remained lifted. Everything from the young woman to the other students, many of whom I might've never seen again, felt like perfect fate.

"Dan!" That following day, a teacher yelled after me in the halls. "I heard you had a good talk with one of our students?"

"I had a nice chat with so many," I said, unsure with whom I was speaking, though her face looked familiar. "And I hope that I helped."

"You more than helped, Dan." She reached out and placed a hand on my shoulder. "I have that young girl in my physiology class, and she confided to me this morning that she had been considering suicide."

Suicide. The word washed over me like a tsunami, rushing a hot wave of emotion to my face, each breath pulsating in my ears.

"Are you okay?"

Her question brought me back. "I-I had no idea."

My journey had touched another and at a time of severe crisis! And, just like the men at the bus station, or the students that high-fived me in the hallways, this troubled young lady had reached out, looking to me for hope.

What if I had not said what she needed to hear?

A worry escalated, turning my stomach. We were talking *suicide*, a choice that cannot be undone. And on more than one occasion, I too had longed for death, but never by my own hand. Nevertheless, the idea that one's darkness could be so deep shook me, forcing me to reconsider my own understanding of despair, which, in turn, fueled my determination to share my love and support to all that need it.

I had found my purpose. It had taken a 400-pound gain for me to see what a wasted life looked like. I had lived through this nightmare and survived. And it was on this day, the day after my first classroom lecture, when I decided to write the book that rests in your hands. And with that revelation came the memory of a pretty author that I had seen in Memphis.

Patricia Garber, Elvis fan, clever conversationalist.

Everybody loves her. I vowed to find out why.

CHAPTER ELEVEN

LOVE YOURSELF

*I may not change the world, but I can change
how I view it!*
~ Journal entry, 2012

ON A BRIGHT SUNDAY, I ASKED to speak with Pastor Rick. He accepted with an air of concern, and I explained how I needed to discuss my marriage. And not with just anyone but someone who would give biblical and ethical advice. At this point, I had heard the opinions of friends—everything from divorce to separation, to *play the field and see what happens.* Now I needed someone who did not know Renee nor formed an opinion before hearing about our unique situation. I was not seeking justice but rather careful wisdom.

Seated in front of Rick's expansive mahogany desk, I was perspiring from a nervousness that matched pre-lecture jitters. Yet, while Rick's frame looked small from behind the solid timber, his spirit was immense and comforting.

"Tell me, Dan, what's on your mind?" His warm smile put me at ease.

"It's my marriage," I began, and for the next hour, we talked about the sad circumstances that had led Renee and me down our current path.

He asked about counseling, and I confided that Renee would not partake, as that had been discussed many years ago, to no avail. And if I were honest, I was long past that option myself.

"You know, Dan, God does not like divorce."

As Rick spoke, my heart felt like fractured glass, just one crack closer to a shatter.

"He grieves greatly over every failed marriage."

I was nodding, unsure of his direction but believing in its importance.

"Infidelity is grounds for divorce, under the eyes of the church and God." He stood up, and the sudden movement heightened my interest. "But I want you to go home, and talk to Renee, one last time. Make sure you have tried everything. Then, if you choose to walk away, God will be with you."

Renee and I were divorced in the fall. And I celebrated Christmas with my mother and siblings in a newly-rented one-bedroom house, two blocks from where I had grown up. The dissolution of my marriage hung over the holiday like a gift nobody wanted to open; we just kept passing it around, speaking off-handedly when the subject came up.

"Has anyone checked in with Renee?" I asked, worried about her first holiday alone. "She isn't taking my calls."

"I did," my mother chimed in. "She hadn't decided where to spend Christmas."

"Mom and I dropped her gifts off," my sister, Crystal, added.

My family had not known of our troubles, and the news of our divorce hit them hard. The timing was tricky for everyone, especially for Renee, as she was not close with her family. But to my family's credit, they reached out to her, sending love as the Hawthorne family does, in patience and kindness. And for that, I was thankful.

Renee has since remarried, and I must admit, to a man much more suited to her. He gets her where I did not, and I am genuinely happy for them both. Sometimes life has a way of righting itself, healing the wrongs, and moving people down more comfortable paths.

While we both deserved a fairytale ending, I was still waiting for mine.

Compartmentalizing kept me on track. I had my life at the gym and the new supportive friends there. I now lived three blocks from my childhood home, where great memories awaited every corner. And at night, I walked, passing the front porch where my mother and father had once sat. Where they watched the neighborhood, discussing concerns, as I joyously played in the yard at dusk. Young and so enamored with life, I never heard these adult conversations, and now, only their presence is remembered.

Though I had lived in the south end my entire life, everything looked new. The roads were freshly paved. Streetlights popped up where once there had been none. Convenient stores that I frequented for chocolate milk were now duplexes! Everything old was new, including me. And charged with all this new energy, I turned to a new social media craze for socialization.

Up to this point, I knew little, only that it was a way to reconnect with old friends while also making new ones. And where I had once spent hours chatting in newsrooms (the chat groups of the times) I joined new groups and made friends quickly. To laugh again was a great gift.

Charting a 200-pound loss, I reached out to others struggling with obesity. And before I knew it, I was confessing to complete strangers. "I used to sneak extra value meals, and then claim it was for my wife." I would laugh while typing the words. "Man, I couldn't even get up off the couch!"

I could not believe the humiliating things I was openly admitting to. But for me, sharing was like therapy, uplifting and unburdening to my soul. I was healing, and judging by the comments from others, they were inspired as well. I was finally an interacting part of humanity. The more I shared, the more people listened. And before I knew it, my understanding of Dan Hawthorne began to change.

I am a good man.

The feeling snuck up on me. I could finally see that carefree boy who only wanted a simple life of toys and fun. And the young man lost to a world that measured success against one's financial worth needed compassion and not disappointment. To go from hate to acceptance was a miracle. And in fact, how I had come to this revelation only became apparent as I prepared for this book. When I realized my recovery had a clearly charted path.

1. Once I cared enough about Dan, only then could I turn my inner key and start my journey. In turn, I cannot turn the key for others. But because you are reading this book, I would say you are well on the path to finding your own way.

2. To succeed, I had to stay focused on the importance of self-care. There was a reason for why I became obese, and to discover it, I journaled daily. I wrote out the bad and the good, using a reaffirming and positive method, like a daily list of my 5 loveable traits. This was not easy, but done every day, I could soon write those affirmations without thought.

3. What makes Dan happy? I spent each week accomplishing something that made my soul smile. It did not have to be big; often, it was a walk in the park, relaxing with an Elvis album, or attempting a new healthy recipe. The only requirement was to focus on myself, my wants, and my needs. And when I gave myself permission to take care of Dan, I felt less like a hamster stuck on a wheel and more like a man with a clear direction. I was a better person all around — not just running, always running.

4. Take baby steps. I celebrated the effort as much as the accomplishment. My spirit was uplifted the day I shopped for clothes in racks that I had never dared to consider! Size 60 went to 55, then 55 to 45, and before I knew it, size 42 had ejected me from the "big-and-tall" section to the "regular" one. And I was never happier than to be a "regular man."

5. Give back. Because helping others cultivates a thankfulness that feeds the soul, I said yes to the offers that came my way.

Dan, can you speak at our church next week?" Of course, the answer was always yes. "Dan, we'd like to have you in front of our seniors." Yes, and yes. The offers came in from all ends of Maryland, from the coast to the big city of Baltimore. And consistently, after a night of giving, I would chart the five things I was most thankful for, which had often happened in the hours prior.

It felt much like courting when my process started, only I was wooing Dan. Am I a caring person? Is my heart in the right place. Do I try my best? And when the answers were always a yes, I began to reconsider the man in the mirror. Maybe, I had been wrong about him; he did deserve to be happy, even at 650 pounds. Even if my sole function were to flash a smile, or pass a hello to a stranger, be a light of kindness in someone's dark place, I could have done that if only I had seen my value.

It is true what they say, a smile is a contagious gift. And when laughing, I would catch a glimpse of the old me, happily connecting with another. I was raised to believe that we are never closer to our created purpose than when we love others. And if we were not designed to be closed off, then starting my recovery by giving love away made sense.

For example, maybe you care deeply for the elderly in your community or have a tender spot for children. Then find a way to help. Do not wait to lose weight first, do it now. All who struggle need a spiritual boost to tackle the rough road ahead. Our emotional condition needs mending to withstand the battle. And when we know our importance, believe in our values, and recognize our qualities, then we will see the life we deserve in front of us. We can see a good person who deserves our time and respect.

I am a natural giver, the type that likes for others to pick a restaurant or a movie. And while putting others first makes me happy, I now understand that I must include myself in this care habit. I encourage everyone to start now; make a list, and write down what you need for yourself. Maybe it's personal time—10 minutes a day, maybe more. If you have children, it could be less, but incorporate it in the weeks ahead, whatever time you need. I promise, regret will not be the word you use when telling others about the blessing.

***

The importance of finding a way together was never more real than when asked by a journalist, to whom did I accredit my success? And I quickly answered Thomas, my friend and instructor at Hagerstown Community College. But not everyone has a Thomas, I realized, and thus began to consider others less fortunate, struggling to find their way alone. When concern sparked bravery, I wrote to Patricia Garber, the author, who, lucky for me, was also a member of Elvis International Fan Club, and easily reached.

Fate or luck? Only the future could say.

She answered me back, quick and easy. For some reason, I thought it would take months; maybe because authors are busier than most people? I did not know. But I was never more pleased than when her return email arrived—warm and friendly, and exhibiting a desire to hear my story. And when she requested a chat over Skype, I jumped at the chance to partake.

For months, I had been stalking her posts online. If I'm honest, I was captivated from the start—back then, in Memphis of 2010. That's when an unfortunate sad man (me) watched an angel from afar. And now, after two years of casual online conversation, we were finally going to chat in person, just the two of us.

When the day came, I was as nervous as an atheist in church. I sat in front of the computer embarrassingly early, focused on the time, and glued to every passing second until the video call came, when I jumped to the answer button.

"Hey, hey, hey." I sounded off like a Saturday morning cartoon.

"Hello," Patricia chuckled. "Nice to meet you, Daniel."

She looked comfortable, sitting in a leather recliner chair, a quilted blanket across her lap, in what I assumed was a home office. Tall evergreens were lurking out the window behind her—a grandiose witness to our first encounter.

"Please call me Dan," I said, admiring a photo of Elvis that hung on the wall beside her. The personal connection allowed me to settle. We were just two Elvis fans chatting; it was that simple.

"Okay, *Dan*," she emphasized, and with a warm smile asked, "I hear you've been on a journey. Why don't you tell me about it?"

The next few hours slipped by like a well-planned vacation, easily rewarding. The conversation was effortless; we talked about the details at the bottom of my existence and my desire to help others with unhealthy food relationships. Soon, our chat turned casual, and the subjects ranged from music to our families and funny childhood stories. The pretty author did not ask too many questions, but much laughter was happening, which I felt was a good sign.

"So, tell me, how does one find an author?" I steered us back to the subject at hand.

"Well, first, you need to get your story organized to paper. Journal it out." She leaned in closer, her porcelain-like features dominating the video screen. "Whoever you get will probably ask you to start there, wanting to see your own words."

My heart sank. "Oh, I see. So, you're not available?"

"Well, Dan, I write fiction. I make up my worlds." Her smile was wide and bright, and my heart skipped like a kid on Christmas Eve.

Get a hold of yourself, I thought, then I heard her say, "What you need is a writer who specializes in Memoir or Self-Help."

While I nodded in agreement, I was pondering the mystery of her eye color; were they blue or green?

"I think you have a story worth telling." She reclaimed my attention. "And once you get the sentiments written out, I'd be happy to help you find someone."

When the session ended, I sat there, flooded with a mix of confusion and thrill. I did not gain an author, but this woman gave me a charge like a defibrillator to the soul. I could feel my heartbeat across my skin, pulsating along my neck, over my wrist. This woman was foreign, scary, and fabulous!

CHAPTER TWELVE

GET COOKING

"What is the secret to cooking rice? Someone please tell me!"
~ Journal entry, 2012

PEOPLE WITH FOOD RELATIONSHIPS, ABOVE all else, are concerned about what they cannot eat when attempting a change. Therefore, from the start, I never asked, "What *can* I eat?" But rather, "What can I *not* eat?" weighed heavily on my mind. The dread of a food change caused me great stress. And I believe this is to be completely normal.

Nobody says, "I cannot wait to have some broccoli; bring it on!"

For me, losing my favorite foods was like grieving a special relationship; what was missing was far more prevalent, even above my own health. And many times,

GET COOKING

I did question my choice of chocolate over life, realizing I was continuously eating sweets right to the grave! But the fear of change kept me from taking that first step of commitment. I did not want to give up soda, I liked cheese, and I felt the whole mess was a drag.

At first, I simply didn't want to do the work. I longed for the fat to just go away, to wake up, like from a dream, and find myself healthy and fit. Then the question, "When can I eat ice cream?" came next.

Food anxiety is natural, it has legs, and it breathes. To an average person, canceling out sweets for a few months is a temporary inconvenience, one they can work around, like switching from gummy bears to gum. No biggie! Most people do not use bagged treats as an emotional crutch; they will not be sabotaged by the fear before a change can even be seen. But to me, the whole sweet saga was a drama that rivaled anything seen on TV.

"You need to give up your chocolate milk habit, Dan, at least for a while," Thomas said while standing over me supporting a bar full of weights.

For two seconds, my mind set to panic. "Why? I'm still losing weight, and it's low fat!"

"Is it sugar-free?" he countered with a frown.

"No, sugar-free is gross!" Instantly, I was 10 again. "I'd rather not bother."

"You're slowing at the scale; give it up for a while," he pleaded. "A time will come when you can enjoy it without limitations."

There was so much to learn. So, I arrived early to Thomas's health and wellness class, a good thirty minutes before the time he had allotted for when I should share my story, just so I could hear the expert advice firsthand. I took notes, writing down every word; rather than white bread, choose multigrain, and the same for pasta. Switch from canned to fresh or frozen vegetables; avoid the preservatives while gaining good nutrition.

Every word made sense; the information was accessible, and in such abundance, I hurriedly scribbled to keep up, asking myself, *Why had I not understood this before?*

"Make sure to get a good balance of all food groups," Thomas said, such as lean protein, veggies, and fruit, no less than three times a day.

Yes! He had mentioned this before, saying, "Your plate should be colorful."

"Three meals and one or two small snacks a day," Thomas added. "And consume lots of water. Don't let yourself get thirsty."

Sugary soda was out, and H2O and I had become one. While Thomas had been guiding me for months, and I questioned almost nothing (chocolate milk debates aside), these were the changes, combined with exercise, that started my weight-loss story. Everything he was telling his class, I could physically prove worked! I WANTED TO JUMP UP and scream, "Look, look, he's right!"

From then on, I asked questions, absorbing everything Thomas told me, and I began to see the food challenge was to think outside the box. Whatever the meal, I made sure it was easy to cook, suited my taste, and was full of colors like red strawberries and green asparagus.

When I first started, I had believed everything, so-called *good* for you, was unpleasing to the palate. So I bucked at the idea of broccoli, clumping warm cheese on the dreaded vegetable to eat it. Brussels sprouts were even worse! I was sure they came from a special place in Hell, cooked by the devil himself.

Who the heck even eats this green monster of the garden?

I never could cook them right—too soft, too hard; the struggle was real. The same was true for those nut-family delights. So at first, it was an effort to eat cashews and almonds instead of chips and crackers. Then I realized I like nuts. It was a switch from the good ole days when I only ate an almond in a chocolate bar.

Soon, my grocery routine changed, and I learned how to avoid the middle aisles of a food store, as they mainly held boxed and canned items. And while I was supposed to be consuming only fresh foods, I had been cooking from a box for so long, I was utterly lost without these easy-to-cook options!

"Can you help me, ma'am?" I stopped a woman near the tangerines. She had three kids in tow and was still smiling, so I figured her a saint. "Do you know where I can find spinach?"

She turned and warmed me with a smile. "Sure, you'll find some bags in the frozen section, aisle four, I think."

"Oh, I'm sorry, but I meant fresh. I've walked up and down, but really, I don't know what it looks like."

"Bless your heart," she cooed, and then walked me to a section and pointed to leafy items tied in a bunch.

I'm going to starve, was my thought while I peered at the fresh produce like it was a threat to life. I'd spent so much time in the cereal aisle that the even word *produce* was foreign to me. I once even looked up its meaning, convinced it was something diabolical. However, sticking to the outside aisles in those early months helped keep the temptations away, especially during the holidays.

Well into my reconditioning, I continued to stroll the candy aisle, looking more out of curiosity, like window shopping on Fifth Avenue. *I am not really going to buy anything; I just want to smell the candy.* To this day, the middle aisles serve as a reminder of why I became obese, why sugar and processed foods fuel diabetes, and why I still only travel the inside corridors for a few needed condiments, like coffee or tea.

Get Cooking

Before my journey began, my food experiences were confined to the family dinner table of 1975. That meant that if the dish had never made it to my mother's table, then I was sure it was undesirable. Furthermore, I understood only what my family consumed, where vegetables came from a can and the meat was spread over toast. Therefore, if the package was unfamiliar, I was skeptical. And I did not understand how to cook it, so the learning curve was steep and wide. But I had to do the work if I wanted the results.

Twenty-four months had passed before fresh foods out-favored a drive-thru. And these newly enjoyed foods were like new friends, the kind you meet and at first find strange. Then the more they are around, you begin to appreciate what makes them different. And the next thing I knew, I was experiencing new foods from all corners of the world.

Now that's a food relationship I could get behind!

Thomas used to say, "What goes in a car's engine directly affects the performance." And harmful gas and cheap oil will have a vehicle as finetuned as a lawnmower. The same was true for my body. When I hit the fast-food eateries, consuming processed foods, I suffered from heartburn and little energy. I was in pain from muscle inflammation and colon trouble, all caused by an overindulgence of carbohydrates. And I quickly became a master at a sugar nap, often falling asleep at a traffic stop!

Some mornings, aware that a treadmill was in my future, I would eat chicken breast from the night before, strawberries, and a healthy carbohydrate, all consumed before hitting the road. When bored, breakfast could be lunch, and lunch maybe a snack.

"Boss, I eat right all day, but around midnight, I'm still hungry." The food monotony had increased, challenging my patience.

"Your body doesn't care what time it is. Eat if you're hungry," Thomas explained. "Just watch your portions and don't eat ice cream!"

Don't eat ice cream? Would these be my famous last words?

If food was life, then the gym was where I went to dream. Where I felt invincible as if I had conquered the worst the world could offer, and only the best of life lay ahead. The challenges at the gym motivated me, like striving to move an extra ten pounds or cycling faster and longer than before. Where I once could barely walk, I now trekked laps around the school's track when the weather was good. I cycled indoors and out, five miles without much effort. So, one can see how defeating the obstacles was an outstanding achievement for a man who once could barely get off the couch.

But of all my misconceptions about keeping fit, my most significant misunderstanding was that exercise was only done indoors. And now that I lived on the south side of Hagerstown, I was a hop-skip from the grocery store, the library, the park. So, on a whim, I parked my car and rode everywhere! I cycled for groceries. I rode the two miles—one each way—to the library, where I worked hard to organize the book you now hold in your hands.

"You rode to the library?" Patricia's laugh left me warm and sappy, like a middle school crush.

That voice should be on the radio, my thoughts briefly roamed. "What, you don't ride?" I asked, shifting on a wobbly library chair.

"Well, my library is over twenty miles away, so no," she said, curiously watching me switch to another chair and yet another. "Listen, you know when I said that I could help you find a writer?"

My attention snapped to the screen.

"I cannot seem to get your story out of my mind. I'm even dreaming about it." Her focus drifted off video, lingering in thought before settling back to me. "This is going to sound crazy."

"I believe in the power of dreams." My heart fluttered with hopeful anticipation. "So, please continue."

"I think we're often guided, if we're listening." She hesitated as if to carefully consider her next words. "And I believe God wants me to help you write your story."

My mind skipped, uncertain of what I'd heard. But when Patricia reclined in the chair, her features softening, awaiting my response, I snapped straight.

"That's great!" I almost jumped into the air, and if she had been with me, I would have hugged her. "When can we start?"

I had been in the same room with Patricia only once—Memphis, 2010. And even then, we had not spoken. So now a plan was needed, one that included travel to the East Coast. She needed to see my world, she said, and hear the stories firsthand. She talked about writing with what she called "all five senses." And I failed to tell her I had no idea what that meant but was anxious to learn. Meanwhile, I was to continue to journal, and as she put it, "Keep yourself positive."

"Will you be alone?" I was curious about her husband.

Her response was quick. "It will just be me."

That evening, I cycled my bike home on remote like a homing pigeon. Hagerstown was the backdrop to my life; its damp streets and alleyways were in my DNA. I cycled a few blocks, slowing at the city park to watch the Tundra swans floating in peaceful pairs.

Are they lovers or friends? I pondered, while a March sun slipped under a pink horizon, and one by one, the streetlamps flashed on—my cue to head home.

The home was lonely. I am not a man that enjoys his own company. I had spent far too many years alone, even though I was married. And now, with nobody to share a meal, no one with whom to inquire about the day, I was left off-balance. Not ready to face a vacant home, I took the long way, once again spinning down Pope Avenue, past my childhood home, coming to a pause at mailbox 1240.

The old house was dark. No kitchen light glowed; the two-story farmhouse looked as lonely as I felt. As I glanced around the neighborhood, I took notice that not a soul sat on the porches of these fine homes. As a child, I remember my mother visiting from each porch, chatting with other parents, no doubt discussing the neighborhood gossip in peace.

Life was simpler then; when that which mattered most revolved around family, friends, and faith. And on this night, while I sat astride my bicycle under a darkening sky, my thoughts drifted to Aunt Thelma. Though she had long ago passed, I remember watching *Planet of the Apes*, my head in her lap, and her caressing my hair until I was fast asleep. My memories came alive on this night, sparked by loneliness—a sentiment I feared would be around for some time to come.

When my memories were exhausted, I turned and headed to my new home, my bachelor pad up the road. I sat on my tiny porch, not ready to go inside. A cat sat on the kitchen window seal, its paw stroking the glass as if to ask, *Why are you out there alone when we await you inside?* I smiled, the feeling of love warming me, even if only from a feline. And when I finally entered my home, three sets of furry feet ran to greet me. I offered each a share of attention, my mood lightening with every caress.

I'm officially the cat-dude next door! And that's okay...

***

I scheduled a speaking engagement on Patricia's first visit. I had spoken at South High, my alma mater, a few times, stressing to the youth, "We all have a purpose; no matter the age, nobody is created for failure." And now that I was focusing on giving back, the event was a perfect place to show Patricia where I wanted to take my story, how people of all ages need positivity in their life.

There is no better place to reach young minds than one's local high school. And Thomas, who also shares a mutual passion for educating our youth, decided to join me. So we set up a demonstration, which highlighted my story with Thomas's expert advice, and set out to make a difference.

I had been conversing with Patricia about this event, excited to show her where I went to school, where my downfall began, and of course, the positives of getting my life back. Looking back, I can see I was much like a teenager on a first date, counting down the hours and minutes until the West Coast plane touched down in the East.

Of course, all my excitement was misplaced. Patricia was married. And judging by the gorgeous log cabin she lived in, I assumed, happily married. Second, I wasn't sure where all this built-up excitement was steaming from, loneliness or project jitters? But I had no desire to mess with the balance of her life, so I vowed to be on my best behavior.

Patricia took a non-stop flight from Portland, Oregon, and arrived in Maryland early evening, in time for the next day's events. While waiting for her in the baggage claim of Baltimore Airport, I went over the plan. My mission? To escort her directly to the hotel for a good night's rest before tomorrow's big event.

She spotted me first, waving a hand to gain my attention. She looked as I imagined an author would—clever, and with her blonde hair pinned up and a pair of gold rim glasses, the song "Hot for Teacher" sprung to mind. Inappropriate, I admit, but it's the curse of all radio DJs that song tracks randomly intrude, and often with little tack.

Like music in motion, she strolled my way. She did not look as if she'd just flown 6 hours. She wasn't dressed like the other passengers, as if they'd stepped out of bed, complete with slippers. Patricia had on black jeans and brown, knee-high boots, a nice mix of professional and casual. But it was her smile that grabbed me, big and welcoming.

"Mr. Dan." Her greeting was both formal and friendly.

"That's Lieutenant Dan to you," I quipped in my best Forest Gump impression while sharing a light hug, consistent with our easy-going banter. "Here, let me take your luggage." I reached for the small bag by her side and was pleased when she allowed me the chivalry.

"Nice and quiet airport," she noted. "Just how I like it."

"Nice to know we're ranking high."

One of Patricia's personal tidbits was that, while she wrote books, she had worked for a major airline since high school. Her life sounded adventurous to someone who had only left Maryland twice, visiting Memphis and Charlotte.

"Your little airport is cute," she quipped, motioning for me to lead the way.

In-person, she sparked with an in-charge persona that intrigued me, and I inwardly chuckled over a thought, one that suggested she was only following because she was not familiar with my car.

While I loaded the bags in the trunk, she sat in the passenger seat. And because the drive to Hagerstown would take an hour, I was already planning our conversation. So first, I chatted randomly about Maryland's history, asking questions to gauge her knowledge and pleased when she showed an interest, which allowed for an extensive range of topics.

"The drive home is more scenic in the daytime," I said, aware that the night's sky would cover Maryland's beautiful views. "Hagerstown's in a valley, right over those mountains up ahead."

Patricia leaned closer to the windshield. "Where's the mountain?"

The car's cab was dark and shadows muddled my view, but I thought I saw her smirking.

"Are you making fun of our mountains?" I playfully huffed, adding, "It may not be the Cascade Mountains, but it's ours, and they're cute!"

"Well, I'm sure they'll look bigger in the morning." She gave my shoulder a pat, and we both laughed.

It felt good to share in a simple conversation outside the gym. I did not want to drop Patricia off; I wanted an all-night cafe where we could talk until dawn. I wanted to feel alive and connected with another human being. But it was October, cold and damp, so we hurried from the car to the hotel, me toting her luggage. And while she signed the guest papers for her stay, I waited, formulating a way to prolong her departure.

Get a grip man, I thought, while catching a glimmer of the ring on her left hand. *Don't act a fool*, I was reminding myself when Patricia spun around, her sudden movement sparking my on-air voice, the one I use when I'm late for a commercial break.

"Alright then, it's a go for tomorrow, all's good and I won't be late." I wheeled her bag to her side. *And we'll be right back after this commercial break.*

"Okay," she said. Then hesitated before adding, "See you at 8 AM?"

"Absolutely." I was aware my voice was still loud, but I found it humorous. So when she reached the elevator, I added louder still, "I'll be here with bells on!"

She glanced back to me, her eyebrows now drawn together in a question over those green—or were they blue?—eyes. When the elevator door opened, I smiled to myself. Then, as she stepped inside, I inwardly laughed, aware she must be wondering what alien planet I had come from. And when the door closed, it did so with a finality that rattled my nerves.

Chapter Thirteen

Give back

"I do not wish away one day of suffering; the pain has made me who I am."
~ Journal entry, 2012

I SHOWED UP WITH COFFEE in hand the following day, smartly dressed in a derby hat, blue jeans, and a collared shirt. And because I had no idea what kind of coffee Patricia might enjoy, I had four cups to choose from. I figured I'd give away whatever she rejected, earning points on foresight and punctuality.

"She is coming, my friend," announced a slight man with a name tag that read *Yash*. His eyes followed me from behind the hotel's check-in desk as I took a seat to wait.

"Thank you for calling her room," I returned.

"You're a very happy man, my friend, very happy indeed," he said in a sing-song accent, offering me a grin that Europeans would call cheeky.

And while I was fishing for a quirky return, Yash held up a newspaper. "This is you, yes?" He pointed to my face on the front cover.

There I was, a full-length picture of a 350-pound me, with a photo of the 650-pound Dan beside it for comparison. Behind the counter, my new friend began to clap his hands. I was so distracted by Patricia's arrival, I had forgotten about *The Herald Mail* news article due out that day.

"Yes, that's me, "I said, blushing while now understanding why Yash felt I was a lucky man.

When the elevator door dinged, our laughter silenced, and out walked my guest for the day. Patricia looked even more elegant than the night before, her blonde hair now down in long ringlets flowing over her shoulders.

As if the moment was a movie, Yash and I locked eyes, and once again, he chimed, "Very lucky, my friend, very lucky," and I pointed to him in a sign of mutual understanding.

"Who's lucky?" Patricia asked, unknowingly interrupting a man-moment.

"We are! The sun is bright, and I have coffee," I recovered, offering the cups to my VIP.

"Perfect," she said and considered my load.

"I didn't know how you liked it." I pointed to the first cup. "So there's sugar, no cream, and then cream and sugar, and of course, sweet cream."

"You, sir, are a man after my own heart."

As Patricia took the sweet cream, I made a mental note and then handed the extras to Yash, whose curious gaze followed us to the exit. Then, with little time to spare, I politely agreed to a drive-thru for breakfast. And while waiting, my stomach flipped, both from pre-lecture jitters and the smell of grease.

"Did you know there are enough calories in that egg sandwich to replace your next three meals?" I threw out the trivia while my hungry passenger consumed her breakfast next to me.

"Don't worry, I'll eat healthy at lunch," she said, and then offered me a crumbling biscuit.

"No, thanks." I laughed. "Been there, done that."

And we all know how that turned out.

The five-mile drive to Hagerstown South High was full of light conversation and humor, which continued until I pulled my green Chrysler (the beast) up to the brick building where I had spent my formative years. I thought how exhilarating it felt to park in the marked space, like breaking the rules with permission. And I snickered as I looked out the back window, gauging how close I was to a parking post, the same pole I'd once tied my friend Barney to, drunk and in his underwear.

Give back

"What's so funny?"

Though Patricia chuckled in compliance. "So many stories, and not enough time," was all the explanation time allowed.

School security was tight, so we waited while our identification was confirmed. The halls were lined with banners announcing an up-and-coming football game, like in the old days. 30 plus years had passed, and I felt like a giant inside the halls that once filled my world. Sports is big in Hagerstown, and though I only played one year of football at South High, I still attend the games, as do most of my friends. Though no one has kids on the field, school pride is alive.

Thomas was waiting in the auditorium, and when we entered, I noticed he had already rallied up a few school athletes to help with the exercise skits we had planned. The goal was to show examples of the exercises students could perform without a gym while motivating them to create healthy food habits. Or, at the very least, put the fear of "this can happen to you" within them, shocking them with *before* photos. And believe me, the picture of a bloated me can scare anybody sober.

After a few introductions, Patricia took a seat in the back. She sat away from the action, preferring to witness the event from a student's perspective. As the students entered the auditorium, I watched the crowd, looking for the quiet and withdrawn teens who needed to hear what I had to say.

The pattern was the same whenever Thomas and I did these events. The athletes sat up front, close to Thomas. He looked like a football coach in khaki pants and a dark polo shirt, rallying the team for a pregame chat. And my targeted teens liked to sit in the back, as far removed as possible, and often prodded forward from a well-intentioned teacher.

"Good morning, South High," Thomas began as a PowerPoint screen flashed on behind him, elevated so all could see.

When the first photo flashed—me at 650 pounds—a whisper buzzed around the room. As curious teens leaned over padded concert seats, vying for a better look, their gaze shifted from me then back to the photo. We allowed the students time before introducing me as the man in the picture. And while they were tackling the contradictions, it's then that I looked to Patricia, happy to see her smiling, clearly keen on the path we'd laid out.

"The man in this picture is Dan Hawthorne at 650 pounds, and the man standing before you is also Dan Hawthorne after losing 300 pounds." The room clapped. "My name is Thomas Burge, and we're here to talk to you about exercise, nutrition, and healthy habits that can keep you fit for life."

With that, Thomas handed the program to me. For the next hour, I led the class down memory lane, sharing many sentiments inside this book, pausing over essential points, like making good food relationships now while they were young so that healthy habits would follow them throughout adulthood. I explained how my pattern of comfort-eating, to heal what was broken, only furthered my decline. Instead, I told them, one could forge healthy food habits and exercise routines to relieve stress, instead of eating. I walked them through my mistakes and then opened the floor to questions.

"Mr. Hawthorne, when I ask my parents for healthier meals, they tell me they don't have the time," a teen girl in the back explained.

This was a common question, as today's parents found themselves with busier schedules.

"I don't know your parents, nor their schedule, but let me suggest that you take the initiative and offer to help with the meals." The young lady's eyes widened with a *what, me?* expression. "Check with your parents first, but everyone here today is old enough to offer to help in the kitchen. And if you're allowed to cook, you may then get a say in the meal."

A quizzical murmur spread around the room as they contemplated the idea of cooking for their families, weighing the value in my words.

"My parents say they can't afford special foods." The statement came from a slight young man on the opposite side of the room.

"That's a concern." I walked closer to the student. "But did you know that you can buy a loaf of wheat bread and fresh deli turkey for the same price as a value meal?"

Judging from the laughter in the room, I assumed many had a food delivery app on their cell phones at that very moment.

"And how about a can of carrots, full of preservatives and salt? While one eight-ounce can costs a dollar, you can get a pound of fresh, raw carrots for the same money. That's not only math but common sense!"

While some considered my words seriously, others rolled their eyes with adolescent boredom.

"The point is that with careful planning, one can cook a full dinner and provide the next day's lunch often with the same money spent on a junk meal! And at the same time…" I pointed to the photo of the 650-pound Dan. "You avoid obesity."

Nothing captures people's attention quite like a photo of a man tempting death.

The question of money came up often, no matter the age of the crowd. We must be vigilant and watch for coupons on meats, fruit, and vegetables if necessary. My mother raised a family of six on one income—challenging, even for 1975. But, if it means we must make more time to find the deals, then that's what we must do! The alternative of year-after-year weight gain, achy joints, and low energy is not an option.

***

As we walked out of South High in the late afternoon, a cool breeze pierced my skin like a hundred tiny needles. Though I wore no coat, I felt a warmth of accomplishment. For me, the day had held a greater purpose, a realization that the years I spent suffering had a point. And my anguish was not wasted. Even Patricia walked a tad lighter in the wind, uplifted, I realized, by the excitement that stirred when the students heard there was a writer in their midst. The word "author" drew hopeful dreamers her way, and she enjoyed the attention, judging by her respectful demeanor.

"Do you like tacos?" I inquired once we were back in the car.

Her face lit up. "You said the magic word!"

I steered the green beast towards a locally favored restaurant known for its south-of-the-border cuisine. For me, the day was a free-food day, where restrictions are lifted—within reason—and favorites can be enjoyed.

"I'll take a margarita, on the rocks, with salt." Patricia was ready when our hostess arrived.

"Same," I chimed in.

"Chips and salsa? Guacamole?" the young woman suggested.

And as if on cue, we both answered, "All of it," and then laughed.

"You should stop copying me," Patricia teased.

We laughed and made small talk, sharing stories about our mutual fur-babies. I explained that I was the official cat-dude in the neighborhood, while Patricia admitted to being an overly-obsessed dog-mom. It had been a long time since I had had an easy conversation with a woman. But even out of practice, stories came effortlessly. So it was not hard to be at ease, though I scrutinized my every move. *Don't hog the guacamole, don't make a mess. And whatever you do, Dan, don't plop food onto your new shirt!*

When it was time to order the main dish, ladies went first, and my stomach tightened as I heard Patricia order a chicken burrito, hold the sour cream, and rice and beans on the side.

I quickly rescanned the menu, searching for a food change, when I heard the hostess address me. "And you, sir?"

She turned my way, pencil hovering over the order tablet. And while she waited, I watched as the eraser fluttered, back and forth like a pendulum, taunting me with a come-on-already rhythm.

Under pressure, I caved and said, "Same." Then I let a beat pass before looking up to my dinner partner.

She watched the show with a hint of humor in her eyes.

"I swear I'm not copying you!" I sounded off like a child. "Really, this is exactly how I would have ordered."

Patricia only smirked. "Good, I'm glad you're not trying to impress me with a burrito."

Our joint laughter spilled into the room, disrupting the couple at the table across from us, more interested in their cellphones than each other.

I let out a sigh of relief, feeling more alive at that moment than any I could remember.

"I haven't had someone to laugh with in a long time," I admitted, lifting a glass to hide my blush behind a sip of water.

"Me neither."

While her words suggested a story, I did not ask her to tell it. I had assumed Patricia was happily married, that was, until this moment. And now, unsure, my thoughts began to race with a concern. For I knew too well the anguish of a marriage gone off-track.

"A woman like you should laugh all the time." I was careful to stay in my lane. *Do not pass go, and do not collect 200 dollars.*

"Well, I do have a large family to keep me entertained."

"And by large, you mean?"

"Italian," she volleyed.

"Like *The Godfather*?" I returned.

"No." She covered her laugh with a hand. "More like *Jersey Shore*."

"Aw, reality TV, even more fun."

Dinner lasted two hours, and in between talks of the book, we discussed our similar hobbies, like Elvis Presley, amazed over our mutual admiration. Like how at the age of 10, we recorded Elvis's movies off the TV to a small cassette player, only to relisten in bed at night. *Girl Happy* was her favorite. And predictably, it was mine also.

"I cannot believe you did that too," I said, relaxing back into the chair.

"Of course! What choice did we have? There was no VHS or DVDs."

When the bill came, I slipped cash into the folder and casually glanced at my watch to see another hour had passed.

"I think we better give this table back," I said, noticing a lingering busboy ready for the next task.

"Right!" She began to collect her purse. "I had no idea of the time."

I stood and waited for Patricia to lead the way out, holding the door as she exited. I enjoyed this old-fashioned custom, often practicing the chivalry with all manner of ladies, the old and young alike. The Maryland night was bitter. And I had deciphered it was either the company or the cold that flushed my cheeks. But either way, it sure felt nice. At one point, we both paused to look at the moon, full and magnificent, and I wondered if she too wished the night would never end.

The drive back to the hotel was quiet. And once parked, nobody moved.

"You know there is one thing we have not talked about," Patricia's voice was solemn now, causing me to wonder what might have altered the mood. "You never talk about Renee."

My mind skipped like a needle across a scratchy record.

"If I'm going to tell your story, we are going to have to talk about your marriage," she said, turning to face me. "And I'm sorry if this is a sore subject."

The topic of my marriage was complex, years in the making, and one that I worried would be hard for another woman to see. *Where do I begin?* The question was huge.

"I don't need to know personal details, but I do have questions." Her demeanor shifted from cozy dinner date to professional, forward and concise.

"I don't blame Renee," I began while Patricia watched me, like a cat at a mouse hole. "It was hard, caring for a husband who weighs over 650 pounds, unable to cater to her needs in so many ways."

Her eyelashes fluttered, and though her face was only partially in the moonlight, I was sure I had made her uncomfortable.

"I'm sorry," she said. And after a moment, she added, "For both of you."

"I blame me."

Patricia nodded, her silence encouraging me to continue.

"I didn't feel like a man, and Renee's escapades, well…they didn't help."

She did not speak. Her gaze drifting out the car's window, seemingly lost to the night. "It's difficult when the trust is gone," she suddenly acknowledged.

The admission stunned me. And I turned just in time to see Patricia's eyes moisten with emotion. My breath held as I dared to believe that, somehow, she knew the pain of rejection. How a once hopeful relationship can simply be over. As I questioned who could reject such a woman, my heart sank further. For I would not wish this sadness on anyone.

Who would not cherish this woman? The idea was unthinkable.

Chapter Fourteen

A Journey in Words

"Words that are hard to speak are easily written."
~ Journal entry, 2012

As an early sun fell across my bed, I lay awake, reliving the previous day's adventures and contemplating the mystery of fate. Here I was, a man with a new life, sleeping in a bed full of cats.

This is it, I thought with a chuckle. *So this is what the future holds; a grown man with 3 cats as his only companionship?*

As I pushed a mound of warm fur away from my side, I set my feet to the floor and headed for the shower. I paused at the mirror to consider the thin-faced man. My reflection was still foreign to me, with pronounced cheekbones and a neck. I had not seen my neck in almost 20 years! And yet there it was, a tad saggy but nonetheless visible. I leaned in closer, locking eyes with the handsome, brown-eyed man before me.

"Not too shabby, Mr. Hawthorne."

I slapped my hands together and then paused, waiting for a mental echo. Nothing. No nasty words counteracted the moment; I was alone with my thoughts. And I could not remember if that had ever happened—a time when Beelzebub had missed a chance at, *Dream on, fatso*, or, *You wish, chubby*.

"That's a day for the history books." I grinned, flashing a quick thumbs up to my reflection, before turning to head for the shower. And because the acoustics were fabulous, I sang my way through three bars of *Fools Rush In*, belting, "Wise men say, only fools fall in love," at the top of my lungs.

Later, while happily enjoying my breakfast, I read over Patricia's last emails while three cats watched at my feet. Her note mentioned a need to discuss our contract agreement and to meet her at the hotel by 9 AM. I glanced at my watch and, seeing it was only 8 AM, I happily returned to two eggs over medium and three slices of turkey bacon, well-done.

"You'd like her, you know," I said to the female feline, who was watching with intense, yellow eyes. And when she meowed back, I quickly answered, "Yes, I hear you."

I don't know why, but cat lovers always converse with their felines. I'm not sure if it's because we're afraid of their disapproval or, Lord forbid, rejection. On the other hand, maybe we simply hate to fail them? These were the mysteries I pondered as I raced out the door to my car, quickly finding myself within Patricia's hotel lobby, and this time with only two coffees in hand.

"My friend," said Yash, waving like a friendly neighbor.

"Hello, buddy," I said, placing a hand over my heart and enjoying the slight bow Yash gave in return.

Butterflies fluttered in my stomach as I took a seat, the heaviness pressed in deep like an anvil to my chest. Patricia was to board a plane in less than 12 hours, and I could not understand my anxiety for the life of me. And if I didn't know better, I may have called this moment the saddest moment in my life. But of course, I'd lived through worse, like obesity, and let's not forget lingering death or poverty at its finest.

So, what do I fear? It was not like I would never see her again. *We're working on a book together,* I rationalized. Plans were in full swing for another visit. *And we are friends, not just online acquaintances.* I tried to talk myself down from the anxiety ledge I teetered on, but the weightiness was hard to shake. And while analyzing my feelings, the elevator chimed, and my guest stepped out with a smile as big as Texas.

"What's this, only two coffees?" she teased. "I must be losing my touch.

"Not at all, but if you don't want it." I turned to Yash. "How about some coffee, my friend?"

"Don't you dare give away my joe." Fast on the draw, she snatched the cup from my hand while offering sincere apologies to Yash.

If I could have slowed the day, drawn out the hours, so that one day felt like a week, I would have waved a magic wand. But fairy godfathers don't exist, and with my green monster valet parked, we soon hurried off to our next adventure.

"What would you like to do on your last day?" I asked as I turned my car down Main Street. "Would you like to see the City Park?"

She flashed a grin. "Yes! That's a perfect place to learn how to write."

I chuckled loudly, and with a hint of cynicism, asked, "You do realize that I barely graduated high school, don't you?"

She gave me a knowing smile before lifting the steaming brew, pausing long enough to add, "You'll see," just before her next sip.

Dogwood trees lined Hagerstown City Park on all sides, giving it a lush, woodsy feel—a forest in the middle of a bustling town. On this day, the park looked especially beautiful, highlighted in white, flowering buds and a pond at its center.

For generations, lovers have congregated here for picnics; families take leisurely walks, and kids feed the ducks. In addition, it's known for free concerts and outdoor movies in the summer—easily the pride of Hagerstown. "So should I follow the teacher?" I asked as I parked along the edge of the park, awaiting my first set of instructions before getting out.

"Why not?" Patricia gave a shrug, opened the door, and stepped into a bright day.

I admit, I was curious. Patricia had never been here before, and yet it was I who followed blindly from behind, as if Patricia were the Pied Piper of Hagerstown, and I a mere visitor. But I did so happily, drawn by a faint scent of zesty perfume and blonde hair that glimmered in the sunshine.

"This is perfect," she cooed from under a welcome banner that hung above the bridge.

Before entering, she looked back as if to check my location, and, satisfied, crossed to the other side. As I stepped across the bridge, I purposely took my time, allowing Patricia a moment to soak in the park's beauty. Like the walking path filled with joggers and bikers or the array of ducks foraging along its edges. And when her gaze fell to the stream near her feet, I was at her side. That's when I realized that the day held a great deal of insight, and a chance to benefit from a foreign perspective. For I had grown up enjoying the park but I had not visited it in over 25 years. And now, free of the chains that once kept me homebound, I was ready to truly absorb its beauty.

"What do you think?" I asked. I couldn't wait to share in the insights already glimmering in her eyes. "What can we learn here?"

"Everything!" Her tone was raised. "Let's start here."

When she pointed to a two-person bench and quickly waved to take a seat, I happily complied. And for several minutes, we sat, me watching her, while she observed the world around us. And just as the silence began to challenge my patience, she asked a simple and yet perplexing question.

"What do you feel, Daniel?"

The sound of my formal name evoked Goosebumps across my flesh, and my mind began to circle within itself. Just in case any woman is wondering, men genuinely dislike this kind of questioning! What do we feel, what do we think? We want to hide in a closet; that's what we think! And because I'm not much different, "I'm happy?" was the first answer that came to mind.

"No, I don't mean, what do you feel as a sentiment." Her eyes flashed with an eagerness. "I mean, what do you feel around you?"

I looked about, still not fully understanding. But I wished to be accommodating, so I again stated the obvious. "The sun is warm," I said, lifting my face to the sky, feeling a hint of warmth inside a seasonally cool breeze.

"That is nice." She lifted her chin towards the sun. "And what do you smell?"

Is she serious? Outside of a good meal, or a buddy's lousy joke, nobody had ever asked.

"Uh…" I looked around, hoping to see a half-eaten apple lying on the ground!

No luck.

"Can you smell the evergreen?" she inquired, pointing to a low-growing bush nearby. "How about the tangy mulch?"

She went on, highlighting the flowers and pinecones. And once the foliage was brought into clearer light, the scents suddenly wafted over me. It was as if nature had fanned its perfume, and I wondered how I had managed to miss it. For what had been hidden had been there all along, if only my senses had been finetuned. But now I could smell everything, hear a leaf scrapping the sidewalk, pushed by wind at my feet.

"Yes!" I sounded off, my excitement like a new discovery. "I get it, I understand."

And we laughed like two people who finally understood the riddled end of a bad joke.

"This is the key to good writing." She waved her arms around. "It's in the wind, the scents, and sounds, all the five senses you live in."

"And you want me to write, what?" I was still unsure.

"From here on out, I'd like you to journal using your senses. Give your story life, make it real," she said, while holding out her hand. I took it and felt a quick squeeze of agreement.

I knew what she wanted. And for a man who spent his free time at the gym merely existing, I needed another mountain to climb. I was restless and longed for the next step in my journey—one where words fill pages, and the cover catches the eye. I had never considered myself cultured, never visited an art gallery or the grand museums in Washington, DC, but I had the soul of an artist. I just needed to widen my canvas. Whether behind a microphone or on the pages of a book, I knew I could make her proud.

***

Baltimore blazed at night, and the M&T Stadium could be seen for miles. While parked in cell phone parking at BWI Airport, I wondered which team challenged the Ravens and whether they were winning. What were the team colors under those field lights? And what radio channel carried the game? These were the questions distracting me as I watched a metal airplane climb into the dark sky, wingtips blinking red in the night. Could that be Patricia's plane? It might as well be because my sadness did not require details. It was as abstract as it was real. And no matter how analyzed, there was only one truth—I was alone, again.

After two days of shared meals, laughs, and long conversations, I was headed home to cats. Just me and the fur-kids, and except for the random visits from my mom and the sisters, I was alone. Every day was the same. After the gym, I would write my story, searching for all the colorful details as Patricia wanted. All the while, I was counting the hours to our next Skype session.

72 hours and 30 minutes, to be exact.

Day 1 was much like day 2, and when the weekend came, a visit with friends on a Saturday night for a cold beer at The Corner Pub was welcomed.

"So when's she coming back?" Barney, that friend who I had once tied half-naked to a light post, asked over a shared meat tray.

"Next month. I've got radio and TV interviews in Ocean City, and she wants to be there." I sifted through the platter, looking for hidden meat under the cheese.

"Look who's bartending." I barely noticed when Barney changed the subject. "Didn't we go to school with her?"

I looked up to a faintly familiar face smiling at us from behind the bar, and because I dislike rudeness, I waved. "Yeah, I think so, but I don't remember her name."

Blonde and with soft, round facial features, she was pretty. And if memory served correctly, I once had a big crush on this now handsome woman, as did all the boys. But that was so long ago, and no matter how hard

I tried, my thoughts always returned to my author, my partner, and the only girl on my mind.

"Patricia's hair color is similar," I casually said before returning to a cheese platter and the search for the next perfect bite.

I could feel Barney's eyes watching me, examining and questioning simultaneously.

"What?" I asked, with a hint of irritated teen in my voice.

"Good God, Dan, you *are* in trouble!"

Chapter Fifteen

Dreaming

"Love coming down."
~ **Diary entry, 2013,
the lyrical wisdom of Jerry Chesnut sung
by Elvis Presley, 1976**

I love her. I scribbled the words in a swift and spontaneous journal entry. And then I stared at it, in fantastical bemusement, as if I were watching snowfall in Hawaii.

I had been jotting down random thoughts as a way of gauging my emotion, much like the inkblot test, except the question was not what I saw but rather what I believed. The damage caused by negativity is immense; I knew this was true. So this was a way to be sure negativity did not linger, not even in the dark corners of my psyche.

But when did "love" happen? I pondered, rereading the three words, desperate to pinpoint a beginning as if to explain it away and make it acceptable. *Was it on her first visit or during our first chat?* Did it really matter?

Then, as if a wind blew away the clouds, I realized: I set my heart to Patricia as far back as Memphis, 2010 when, at 650 pounds, I watched an angel float into a banquet room. And now, having spent time with her, encouraged by her spirit, it was evident from where these three words came from. Love was fueled by fascination, cemented by our mutual similarities.

The big problem: Patricia was married. And even if she was available, my marriage had been a trainwreck. And I should have been good at marriage, I considered. I had such notable examples in my parents. Of course, they had their troubles, as all do, but they were great examples of commitment and everlasting love. To quote Oliver Hardy, I thought, *This is a fine mess you've gotten me into, Daniel.*

"Three minutes to go," I said while shifting a sleeping cat away from the keyboard and being screeched at in disapproval. "Sorry, buddy, but I need the space."

I looked around my bedroom, scanning for an unsightly mess. The room was lit by a single bedside lamp, casting shadows to the far corner of the room where I sat. The computer highlighted my face like a sci-fi movie. And I was contemplating how to fix the floating head visual when the call came.

"Hello!" While I took a deep breath to calm my racing heart, I noticed Patricia was not in her office.

She lounged on a brown, leather couch in what I assumed was her living room. The room looked cozy, with golden pine lining the walls, giving off a sense of intimacy.

"Have I seen this room before?" I knew the answer, but the question allowed time to enjoy the view, from the vaulted ceilings to the A-frame windows, and a half-empty glass of wine by her side, as if celebrating the end of a good day.

"No, I don't conduct business out here much," she said, looking around the room with clear admiration in her eyes.

"It's beautiful," I admitted while a ping of curiosity chimed. "Did you have a good writing day?"

"I wrote the introduction today. Would you like to hear it?" she asked, rather nonchalantly.

Would I like a beautiful woman to read from our book? There was nothing I wanted more. And when she began, "I liked myself once…" those first words transported me back; the anguish was so real, I can still feel it in my gut.

"Do you like it?" she asked, and for a moment, I sat wordlessly, the only evidence of life showed on my grinning face.

"Yes! Y-Yes!" I was stammering now. "You really captured me. Did you get this from my journals?"

She said she had, but it was unbelievable that my journaling could derive such sentiments. I felt my written words were sketchy at best, though they'd improved over time. I had tried to write in living color, as she had asked, but this was more than I could have hoped for.

"You know, writing is not just the story. It's also structure, the format, and that's what most new writers struggle with, at first."

"I am so thankful to have you helping me," I said, ready for a virtual celebration, and since Patricia had wine, I ran to the fridge for a cold brew. "Here's to *Getting My Life Back*, or whatever we decide to call it!"

The hours were marked with glasses of wine and bottles of beer, and laughter that echoed over a four-thousand-mile separation that felt more like a neighborhood block. Time worked in Patricia's favor; where it was 11 PM there, it was 2 AM on the East Coast. But time mattered not. I would have stayed up forever.

"Have you worked out the flights East?" I asked.

Patricia was set to join me for radio and TV events in Ocean City, and I was anxious for her to see where the final days of my journey had taken place.

"Almost," she said, shifting to adjust the pillow at her back. "There's drama at Portland Airport, but it should be worked out in time."

When her fidgeting continued, first adjusting a blanket then resting the wine glass to a table, only to pick it up again, I began to wonder. "Is everything okay?" I asked while she petted a dog at her feet.

"I'm getting laid off." She tossed out the news like a weather forecast. *Today we have mostly sunny skies, mixed with long waits in the unemployment line.*

"Excuse me?" I wanted to hear it again.

"I have twenty-five years, but the airline is pulling out of Oregon." Her smile weakened around the edges, and before a man could even prepare for it, a single tear tinkled over the edge.

"Oh, no." I was instantly sober. "And what will happen?"

She drew in a deep breath. "Basically, I will be asked to relocate or quit."

I never wanted to know more about the aviation industry than now, but all I could think of were the obstacles—her home, her family, her husband.

"I am so sorry, Patricia." I was at a loss. "Listen, things always work out. One never knows what's coming next."

I made a point to avoid the typical sentiments, like, "When God closes a door, he opens a window," or, "God never gives you more than you can manage." None of these clichés help; at least, they never did for me. So instead, I search for something tangible, an olive branch one can hang on to.

"Try to focus on something positive, like your writing," I offered, as she wiped away tears with the back of her hand. "Stay busy."

I am not helping, I began to fret.

Face it, some men are ill-equipped for high emotion, and where tears are involved, I am seriously ill-prepared. I also possessed no phone numbers, nor did I know the names of anyone significant in Patricia's life. I couldn't just call and say, "Hey (mom, dad, sister), she's distraught, maybe you should call her."

"I'm even more thankful for our project now." I could hear Patricia's words but could not see her. The dog at her feet had now stood, no doubt to check on the upset human in the room.

"At least a trip East will keep you busy," I suggested, bobbing my head left and right, unable to see around a large dog butt.

I was later told the caring canine's name was Brinkley, a silver-colored Labrador, not more than two years old. And as the only other physical life in the room, I was grateful for his consoling presence. With his chest in her lap, I watched as he tried to lick away the tears, to both protest and eventual laughter. Since childhood, I had not owned a dog, but the care Brinkley bestowed eased my worry; Patricia was not alone after all.

***

The Giant in Me

When I drove across the Bay Bridge that spring, Ocean City Maryland couldn't have looked more poetic with the beautiful Patricia by my side. With mostly sunny skies and enough clouds to mark the horizon, a fluffy, white distinction marked where the sky ends and the sea begins.

"What would you like to see first, Patricia Lee?" I playfully goaded, using her middle name in a friendly but cozy manner.

"You pick, Daniel Wayne." She grinned, switching to the formal for contrast.

I pulled my beast of a car into Sunset Park, allowing Patricia to view the Ocean City Inlet, a channel where the water flows in and out of the Sinepuxent Bay from the Atlantic Ocean. For a moment, we watched the water crash against a series of jetties, exploding a fan of spray that reached my windshield. There was a time when the peninsula was one with the fledgling town of Ocean City, but that was long ago, after the great storm that separated the land into what is now Assateague Island.

"This is the spot." I pointed to people milling about. "I used to come and watch the happy tourists while slowly killing myself with breakfast or lunch number two."

I had left Ocean City in late 2010 a very different man. I had metamorphized from a once-happy dreamer to a man with no ambition.

"I was angry, questioning why a tourist should look so happy," I reminisced, while remorse swelled. I had lived a block from the beach for years, and yet I was oblivious to its beauty.

It was May, and though chilly, I opened the car's windows to let in the salty air. A Ferris wheel known as The Giant Wheel loomed over the pier in the distance. I could hear the echoes of laughter, the bells and whistles that flowed from the arcades and shops along the boardwalk.

Because we had time to spare, I drove Patricia around, pointing out eatery after eatery—all the places where big-me went to self-medicate. Simply speaking, I'd spilled my life's blood all over this town and barely gotten away alive. But it was when Patricia saw the mobile house where I last lived, with its leaning front steps and rusty roofline, that reality sank in.

"Three of you lived in there?" She looked on in wide-eyed wonder. "How in the world…?"

My sentiments exactly. I explained how the outside didn't do the inside justice. It was worse! Little-to-no kitchen, a bathroom far too tiny for a man of my size, and two bedrooms offering zero privacy, even though on opposite ends of the house.

"The sounds that came from our roommate's room…" I cringed. "It would make a prostitute blush."

All nightmares aside, the tiny mobile home had hosted the best moment of my life—the mirror moment. When I had it out with God and myself. When I turned my internal key for the first time, and took back my life.

But why did I eat? That was the question that continued to haunt me.

Even with distractions, like Patricia in the car and a pending media appointment, I constantly worked the puzzle. And if I am honest, the answer had always been about love. Or rather, feeling unloved. It boiled down to the simple fact that once grown and out of the house, life sucked.

And I hated me. The grown Dan was not what I expected, the opposite of what the world said a man should be—successful, strong, a leader. I missed the love and support of young Danny.

"Where did you go?" Patricia interrupted my daydream.

"I was pondering the past," I said, explaining how a meal still takes me back to a time when I had my whole life before me. When I was a happy and cute six-year-old. And as I explained to Patricia about Nan's meatloaf and Aunt Thelma's special treats, I realized I knew why I had become 650 pounds.

"I felt so loved as a child," I admitted, recognizing my desire to feel love, even now. "And I just don't anymore."

High on a rush of honesty, I explained to Patricia how the old me ate to remember a time when I was loved. When loving hands prepared meals, cared for me. And when I was done, my admissions hung in the air, almost tangible.

"Thank you for sharing that with me." Though Patricia's words were soft, it was her hand on my arm that warmed me. "You're a wonderful man, Dan. And you will find love. I know you will."

How did she know? I wanted to ask. And the question remained with me throughout the day, echoing at every appointment, and during each radio interview, like a heckler in the crowd. Will he be loved? When will he find this love?

It was hard to focus with my attentions divided, trying to listen to the interview host while also monitoring Patricia, as she sat close by, me watching her and her watching me. And even when I was not observing, I worried. *Is she comfortable? Does she need water, food maybe? Is she bored?*

Focus, please stay focused.

"Tell me, Dan." The radio host recaptured my attention. "What would you tell people who are struggling right now?"

"I'd say, don't give up, you are worth it." I readjusted in my chair, as a twinge of pain radiated in my lower abdomen. "You are loved. You are important. And you are worth it."

"You heard it here, folks. You are loved, and we love you here too…" The man's voice was like a reverberation, and I barely heard the show's official end.

When I unhooked myself from the headset and began to lift my body, another pain ignited; this time it went around my side and into my back.

"Are you okay?" the host asked, quickly flicking his microphone to the off position.

"I may have lost three hundred and fifty pounds but only a petite woman would fit in that chair!" I teased, successfully easing out of the chair and to my feet.

Everyone laughed. Except me.

"You did great. What a fabulous interview!" Patricia exclaimed as we exited the studio, her excitement obvious as she switched topics, from radio to the difference between West Coast and East Coast sand.

"Our sand is mostly grey, rough on the feet." She spoke while I drove. "But here on the East Coast, it's so light in color and softer too."

I could not speak, as her cheerful words filled every available space in the conversation. It was as if the banter was needed to distract from whatever consumed her mind, so I practiced listening while working hard to not dwell on the cause of that odd and out of place pain.

"Is this a good time to bring up the book contract?" Patricia suddenly switched gears.

And there we have it, I considered, where her mind had been this whole time, consumed with contractual jitters. Patricia carried herself so well; it was fun knowing a confident woman could be nervous about such business formalities.

"Will you be easy on me?" I asked, attentive and ready. "Or will you be my Colonel Tom Parker?"

With that, she tossed her head back and laughed.

"Not exactly." She reached in her purse and retrieved a piece of paper. "But do read this over and tell me if it'll do?"

I never read it. Money didn't matter to me. I would have given her all my royalties, if she'd asked.

Chapter Sixteen

Consequences

"I'm as strong as a horse!"
~ Journal entry, 2013

As Patricia and I cruised down I-97 towards Baltimore, the pain was like a backseat driver—if they were 5 and screaming for attention. I barely noticed the beauty of Charmed City as we passed. Even with all the lights and action, the big city could not compete with the deep ache that now radiated from my belly to my lower back. Perspiration had begun to bead across my forehead, and though I could not be sure, a fever felt imminent.

"Are you okay?" Patricia asked, because no matter how hard men try, women miss nothing.

And in typical man-fashion, I insisted, "I'm fine." And judging by Patricia's glare, she was not convinced.

We were 30 miles outside of Hagerstown when my chills metamorphosed into an uncontrollable all-over body tremor.

"Can I turn up the heat?" My words sounded shaky, even to me, and without waiting for a response, I reached over and flipped the switch to high.

Had my mind been clear, I may have understood that a chilly night in May was not the problem. But I was confused and became more so with every passing mile.

"You really don't look good, Dan." Patricia reached over and placed a palm to my forehead. "You're on fire!"

I looked at her. I could see her mouth was moving, but the words were like a backward sentence in my mind.

"Pull over," she demanded. And without a single complaint, I did as I was told, parking the car on the wide shoulder of I-70.

When I stepped out, the cool of the night skated across my flesh. I paused to enjoy a fleeting moment of relief, but it was gone too soon. The heat of my body engulfed the chill in the evening. And as I walked, my feet were like bricks, scraping the ground with every shuffling step. I took my time, fighting off wave after wave of nausea on my way to the passenger door.

"My house is ten minutes further. Can you just drop me off?" When I spoke, I coughed back the bile that now burned the back of my throat.

Lucky for me, women are trained to ignore the nonsense men say when sick. Whereas, in contradiction, had a buddy been with me on this night, I would have been dropped at home, and the outcome would have been very different. But Patricia's only response was, "No," and then, like a woman on a mission, she reached for my cell phone and opened it to what I assumed was Google Maps.

What happened next remains a blur, as another wave of pain sparked, this time doubling me over in my seat. But I vaguely remember the word *Hospital*, blurred under bright lights and loud voices.

Let me pause here for an important announcement: What we do to our body now *will* haunt us later.

This is not happening, I considered, as I lay sprawled across a hospital gurney, nurses rushing and I-V bags dripping fluids into my body. I was in septic shock, they said. A kidney stone was lodged in my urinary track, unable to pass, and as it sat there, an infection spread. And though my mind was foggy, I understood that I could have died.

"You had an angel tonight." A doctor, young enough to be my son, shared the news. "You wouldn't be with us if your wife hadn't brought you in."

Wife? I smiled, enjoying the sound of that word. I thought about correcting him, but the explanation sounded silly in my head, so I said nothing. The dramatic details of this love-sick man just made me feel sad.

"She's waiting outside. Would you like me to bring her in?" the youthful doctor with the thick hair asked. And while I was reminiscing to a time when I had hair, my angel entered the room and I automatically reached for her.

"Thank you for not taking me home, Patricia Lee." I couldn't express my thanks fast enough, lifting the back of her hand to my lips. "Thank God you were with me. Had you not been with me, I would have gone home to bed."

"And never woke," the young doctor added.

"Thank you, Doc." Gushing with emotion now, either from the drugs, or, I prefer to think, an immense thankfulness, I added, "And I'm grateful to the nurses, too," not wanting to leave anyone out.

Everyone in the room was smiling, laughing, and seemingly enjoying a rare night with a happy ending. Later, they zapped my stones into fine pieces. And, I considered, maybe it was nights like these, when the good outweighed the bad, that lessons were revealed for us all. Before this night, I knew little about my body and even less about its primary function.

I admit I have a tendency to ignore what ails me, figuring that if it's bleeding, slap on a band-aid. And if that doesn't work, try duct tape. So had I been listening to my body, I should have questioned how I felt on those days leading to Patricia's visit. But her arrival and the pending media fun in Ocean City outweighed any discomfort, and I called it "nothing."

After all, I had just seen my doctor. He announced I was healthy, and I did not ask, nor did the doctor mention, any consequence from a drastic change in diet. Like how one's body can create kidney stones in response to the change. Or how, after losing 350 pounds, it's easy to romanticize one's second chance at life, never considering the consequences.

No diabetes lingered. That's all I cared about. My cholesterol and blood pressure were in line. So much had improved; I ignored the more minor clues. And when something did arise, I diagnosed it as gas or indigestion. It sounded simple. I often consumed antacids like candy, and since when had anyone died from gas?

Death by a fart? That I doubted.

***

A day later, I was released from the hospital and home. As I dressed for the day, I stood naked in front of a full-length mirror, for the first time since losing 300 pounds, entirely in the buff. No shower towel, no underwear, nothing to obstruct my view. Naked as a jaybird!

What a mess, I thought, then lifted an arm, watching my reflection.

"Can you believe this?" I looked to the cat at my feet, its head tilted and ears perked. "Yeah, me neither."

Approximately three inches of loose skin hung from my biceps. Extra layers dangled from my legs, chest, underarms, and belly. And when I turned sideways, I scrutinized the amount of unwanted flesh.

I did this. I nodded. *Me, myself, and I have created this vision.* The scars were mine and mine alone. There were options, I knew. But I had investigated the procedure, such as skin removal, and what I found scared me beyond belief.

Do you know that one's skin is the body's largest organ? Because, until this moment, I was not fully aware of the fact. Nor did I understand the cost, the pain, and the probability of the many surgeries for all that skin.

10 percent. I figured that was how much skin needed amputation overall. The act alone may tally a 50-pound weight loss, but could one pound justify the pain?

As I contemplated these facts, my eyes drifted south, and I smiled at the sight of a belly button. I had not seen it without the aid of a mirror in years. And to my shock, what had once been pushed outward was now inward. *The human body is amazing!* I thought, reflecting on the mystery of how it can recover when all seems lost.

As my mood shifted from grim to curious, I continued examining. Finally, I pulled my gaze from my reflection and now viewed the full vision; the resets, the way my ankles rolled outward, bent bones from 650 pounds of pressure. And then, looking closer, I realized the imperfections suggested a bigger picture—a more beautiful story, for they told of struggle and success.

"I better get a move on." I looked down to my little cat, who chirped back in agreement. "A pretty girl is waiting."

I was not 100% when I arrived at the hotel. And after collecting Patricia, I drove to the church, parked, and waited for my nerves to settle. Though I'd shared my story many times before, this gathering was special. For this was the first time that Patricia would read the introduction of our book to a packed house! Nothing could have kept me away, especially not an annoying kidney stone.

An awkwardness circled within our silence. And for the first time, I did not know what to say. Of course, I had already thanked her an embarrassing number of times, but still, it never felt enough. And I was embarrassed—for subjecting her to an emergency room all-nighter, for leaving her to fend for herself in a strange town for over 24 hours. But mostly, I felt guilty for being more interested in our time together rather than my own health and the warning signs.

"Are you sure you're up for this?" she questioned, her eyes scanning mine for the answer she wanted to hear.

"Yes. Thank you." I grimaced over the realization that I had thanked her, yet again. "It's all under control."

We exited the car, and as I walked towards the towering brick building, with a cross perched on its top, excitement filled my chest like bees in a hive. We carried in our arms stacks of inspirational pamphlets. The night air felt charged as if nature were predicting an energizing outcome. The moon was full over our heads, casting a glow so bright, I would have guessed it earlier than 6 o'clock.

"Welcome, Daniel." The parishioner shook my hand when I entered, and then turned to Patricia to add, "We are so happy to have you both here tonight."

The church sanctuary had a homey feel, with plush, beige carpet and sconce lighting along the walls filtering a golden light throughout the room. The rows of dark, mahogany pews were already full of smiling people, and they watched us take our seats down front as instructed. And when the pastor approached the pulpit, the hum of conversation fell silent.

"I am so happy you're here tonight. And we're especially blessed to have a guest, who will be speaking to us about God's love and healing."

As the pastor spoke about the struggle of life and seeking God's grace inside the fight, I tried to focus, but my attention kept drifting to a raised stage, just behind the podium, and a wooden cross nailed to the wall. And I contemplated the symbol of faith and how the pastor was correct; we often fail to see the good inside the darkness.

I admit, for years, doom and gloom were all I could see. But, of course, that did not mean goodness was absent, only that my focus was askew. And I wondered how different my journey could have been had my faith been stronger. Or was that the lesson after all?

"Let's welcome Daniel Hawthorne to the podium." The sound of my name snapped me back to the present.

I sprung to my feet, adrenaline surging. But before I could share, I explained to the crowd that I had a special treat—"A lovely lady who has agreed to lend us her talent." And with that, I asked Patricia to take the stage. Then I went back to my seat, anxious but ready to listen.

Of course, I had read the piece myself, but not with an audience. So, I was happy to see Patricia relaxed behind the podium, the microphone drawn close but not too close. And when the room fell instantly quiet, I imagined all breaths held in expectation like my own.

"I liked myself once..." Patricia began, and as she read on, I heard sniffing at my back, as all listeners became moved by emotion.

Unable to resist, I turned to look at the room. And found all eyes on Patricia, each face flooded with a vast array of expression. My story resonated from sadness to shock, to interest, and even pain. But not strictly for whom I had imagined.

When I scanned the crowd further, I found not one obese soul present, yet there was a display of suffering on each face. And that's when I knew the weight of my story lies in the anguish, the struggle. It's the day after day of swimming against the current, an upstream battle experienced by all human life that moves us; the question of how I managed the darkness resonated. How did I find peace and escape self-destruction? How did I survive?

Without knowing it, I had lived the answer to so many questions—I survived more than obesity. I cultivated a giving heart, a positive mind, and faith.

"I was not just that big guy... I was obese." A flash of applause erupted as Patricia read the last sentence. Goosebumps engulfed my flesh.

Next, it was my turn.

When we passed, Patricia gave me a nod as if to say, *knock 'em dead*. And instantly, I broke out in chills, and my bald scalp tingled. I walked to the stage, weak-kneed as if treading on a trampoline. Then I turned to the crowd and asked, "Do you like the story so far?" And another round of approval commenced.

For 90 minutes, I discussed my journey, pointing out the hills and valleys. I took questions, gave hugs, and in the end, I was an emotional wreck. Even my voice cracked through the toughest of parts, like how it felt to be unloved and alone. Then I drove home the message—nobody is unworthy, we all deserve love, and we must love ourselves first and then pass it on!

Overall, the night was more than a success; it was eye-opening and heart-filling. I felt emotionally and spiritually complete. And when my stomach growled, a reminder of the importance of food, I suggested a celebration with pizza.

"You do realize that dairy contributes to kidney stones?" Patricia chose to share this nugget of helpful information as we exited a favored pizzeria and headed for the car.

I paused behind her, arms hot with extra mozzarella and ham. "Seriously?" I yelled at her back. *Now she tells me!*

When we entered the hotel lobby, Yash greeted us, but we did not stop for conversation. Instead, we headed for Patricia's room and the promise of Fox's pizza.

"This is so good!" I hummed over yet another slice, eyes closed, giving myself over to warm cheese and Italian sauce.

The setting was odd, me at a table near the window, gobbling from an open pie box, while Patricia lounged with two slices on a napkin from the bed. We looked like a pack of hungry wolves, quietly consuming a kill. No eye contact, and few words between the grunts and chewing.

"I may explode," Patricia offered, holding her gut, and I nodded in agreement.

"I used to be able to eat a whole pie." My stomach churned at the thought while Patricia scrunched her nose.

"That's just wrong," she said, and then randomly asked. "How are you feeling?"

"I'm happy," I quipped, circling back with, "how about you, are you happy?"

She looked at me, eyes narrowing, as if suspicious of the motivation behind the question. I didn't know why I asked. I could the worry in her eyes. Between the drama in her life and my hospital event, her visit had lacked animation and the clever retorts I was used to.

"Am I happy?" She chuckled. "Let me count the ways. First, I've given my job twenty-five years, but they don't care. And then my husband, I've given him twenty-four years, and the sentiment is much the same."

When she stopped, her eyes dared a response. And my thoughts were racing around this complex puzzle. The job equation did not surprise me; big corporations suck. They just do. But the relationship factor floored me. What was her husband thinking? Did he not know what he had?

"My job is asking me to move," she quickly added.

"And?" There was more, and I wanted to hear it.

"And if I don't, I will lose my retirement. And if I do, I lose my husband."

The second bit landed like a bomb, my expression amplified by the aftershock.

"You're kidding," I struggled. "Surely he'll go with you?"

"No," she said flatly.

"But, surely…" I was still floundering when she intervened.

"He won't move." Her voice was stern. "He has a job and his own concerns."

This last sentiment echoed with a matter-of-fact end. *What else can I say?* I pondered while the mood in the room went stale, as if the oxygen had been sucked, and we were left with only carbon dioxide and insignificant points.

"Where will you move to then?" I asked the obvious next question.

"I have five choices." She drew in a breath and tucked a blonde hair behind an ear, as if to steady herself. "Texas, New York, Washington DC, Virginia, and Maryland."

Virginia, DC, and Maryland. My mind circled the news like a hungry vulture. I couldn't believe my ears. *This is horrible… Or is it?*

Chapter Seventeen

Confidence

"High above the halls of Hagerstown Community college, welcome to Getting My Life Back, with Dan Hawthorne and The Boss, Thomas Burge."
~ **Monolog, 2013**

"Fitness radio, why not?" was my response when Tim, a fellow radio buff who had heard about me through a mutual friend, asked to air my story over his online fitness channel.

"It's radio, your specialty," he explained.

But rather than music, Tim shared information, about fitness and wellness, yoga and meditation. It was not on the dial but instead on the web. I had no idea what he was talking about, unfamiliar with current trends; the concept was hard to follow. And I hadn't been on the radio for over 5 years. I was old-school, oblivious to the craze of podcasts and YouTubers. But I loved radio and I wanted to learn. So, before I knew it, I was hosting a show every morning, five days a week, from Hagerstown College.

My mentor, Thomas Burge, joined me. He supplied the knowledge, and I was the voice. Together, we shared all things fitness on a show called "Getting My Life Back." Unfortunately, we didn't have a radio studio. So instead, we used the sports booth inside the arena at the college and shared our mutual story. The acoustics were perfect, and by the miracle of laptops and headsets, we linked to Tim's fitness station via the web and talked about health and wellness to millions of listeners.

We switched roles for one hour a day; Thomas, a newbie to broadcasting, became the intern, and I, his teacher. We worked well together. Thomas was a quick study, eager to share the ins and outs of fitness. While I was the average guy, with some gym know-how and a ton of inspiration, Thomas answered the technical questions. I reached people more personally, encouraging a healthy relationship with food. And the combination worked. The show quickly gained popularity, re-kindling my love for broadcasting.

"I still think I'm six hundred and fifty pounds," I told Thomas, speaking more for our listeners, as Thomas had heard it all before. "When I see an obstacle, be it a squat bar or whatever, I immediately assume I cannot do it. The giant cannot do it."

It was early June, when girls and boys alike begin to focus on summer break, and inevitably, their outward appearance. So we highlighted the importance of confidence and how to build it. And what better example than me, a man who once couldn't walk, much less wear a bathing suit?

"But you never gave up, did you?" Thomas added. "How did you rebuild your self-confidence?"

Thomas knew I had his entire staff cheering me on day after day. For the last two years, I've had a gym full of young and old helping to build my courage. When I said *no way*, they said *give it a try*. They were my reality check when my perspective kept changing, an offset from the giant mode to average man settings.

But not everyone has a team, and in looking back, I wonder if I could have prevailed without the support. The question haunts me. And if I'm honest, I know the answer—I needed their support. There is no shame in needing the help of professionals, spouses, friends, and family. My only regret is that I did not reach out earlier, understanding my limitations and the need for assistance.

"Thomas, look, I can cross my legs!" My voice rose with such excitement as if Thomas had never seen the miracle before. But of course, he had.

My body surprised me every day. And on this day, I spoke for 10 minutes on how the giant me once sat, legs pushed wide apart. And how my once-overextended midsection was much like a camel's hump, separating one thigh from the other. And though listeners couldn't see me, I crossed my legs freely and sat like an average man, as if for the first time.

"Trisha Lee, watch this." Later that night, I crossed my legs for the camera, showing Patricia during what had become our nightly Skype session.

"The thrill is real, right?" she said with a coy grin. "You should be proud."

My face warmed with a realization—I was proud, and possibly for the first time.

"I always knew I had a purpose," I spoke, considering the beautiful lady packing up her office, filling box after box of personal belongings.

The vision struck my heart, taking my very breath away. Off-camera, I heard a man speak, asking Patricia if she wanted some item, or this and that. To which she quickly declined. Was that the voice of her husband? Or maybe her brother?

I should hang up. The idea circled, yet I didn't want to leave her.

"Have you picked a city yet?" If she had, she had not told me.

If I was anxious, I couldn't imagine the dread her family was feeling. Patricia and her mother were close, bonded as I had never seen two souls before. And her sister's home was like a second residence. A two-hour drive south to Eugene, Oregon, Patricia could often be found helping with her 14-year-old niece or lending a hand with her sister's new business.

When it was time for Patricia to leave, the loss to that family would be significant.

"I've almost decided," she said, taking a picture from the wall and placing the black frame between sheets of cream paper to fold, once and then twice. "I have to tell them by tomorrow."

As if on cue, the family Labrador I had come to know as Brinkley entered the office, and Patricia's face instantly lit up.

"Come here, buddy-boo," she called out to the dog, bending over and grabbing the tail-wagger by the neck to give him a squeeze. The dog did a little jig in her arms, a happy dance if I had ever seen one. "Now, off you go. Get Mr. Bubble so we don't forget to take him."

With a gentle push, Brinkley raced out of the room like a hound on the hunt, eager to retrieve what I assumed was a favored toy.

"He's coming with you, right?" I gave a knowing chuckle, and Patricia pointed to me as if to say I was on the mark.

***

Two weeks later, my prayers were answered; Patricia had chosen a city. My heart raced as I opened an email with a subject line that said, *Decided,* and then I swiftly scanned through Patricia's words, my eyes pausing over—Virginia. She had been approved to work at Dulles International Airport!

For me, Virginia's Dulles Airport was the same distance as Maryland's Baltimore Airport, so she would be closer, no matter what. And while part of me wanted to celebrate this good fortune, another kept returning to Patricia's family and the fact that the long-distance move would bring much grief.

Has she told everyone? If so, how did it go? The questions kept spinning. And I longed for an update, but outside of singular email correspondence, all had been quiet.

Maybe, I should call? I stared at my phone, lying face down on an end table nearby. An urge to hear her voice swelled. But what could I say? Nothing would make this less painful. And as every day passed without a word from Patricia, I grew more panicky.

She needs more time, I told myself on day three. Time to grieve and gather the strength necessary for what's to come. And while Patricia was a strong woman, I understood she viewed life through the lens of an artist, always looking for a happy ending. And when life left her disappointed, I had watched her analyze the events like a troubling story, red correction pencil handy, ready to cut an entire chapter and begin from scratch.

She's starting over, and I know a little about that. I had always thought The Beatles lyric—"life is what happens while you're busy making other plans"—was a perfect explanation for all of life's mishaps. Because, after all, the *whys* are revealed in the future, not in the now.

"Hello," Patricia finally took my call. Her voice sounded small, like a child begging for a reprieve.

"Hey, it's me. Is this a bad time?" I was mentally giving her a hug.

"No," she said; she was just clearing a closet. And her family was due soon, to help before the movers arrived.

"How is everyone?"

"Good but not great." Her voice cracked, but she caught herself. "Ironically, my niece is handling it better than the adults. I think it hasn't sunk in."

The airline gave her 4 weeks to move her life, to clear a 4-bedroom home, end a marriage, and say goodbye to everyone she cared about—it was unimaginable.

"I cannot think straight, and I have writer's block now too."

What did she just say? Surely, she is not trying to write.

"Maybe you should get another writer. I'm a mess." Her words were racing now, like someone pushed fast forward. "I will give you what's done, all the writing, it's yours."

"Hold up—"

"I can't do it. I don't know when I will be able to do it, and besides…"

"Wait!" When I heard the panic in my voice, I quickly recanted. "I'm sorry, but please, wait a minute."

There was silence on the other end. And for a moment, I worried Patricia had hung up, irritated over the sound of my raised voice or plain frustration. Then a tiny whimper came, and I knew she was listening.

"I don't want anyone else. I want you." I was not below begging, and even in a panic, I realized how love-sick I sounded. "You are meant to share the story; you know me best."

More sniffing could be heard.

"Please, we have time. I'll be here." If I could have yelled, 'Beam me up, Scotty' to anyone with the capability of warp drive, I would have instantly been at her side. "We'll work it out together, okay?"

Agonizing seconds passed until I heard the weak, "Okay," which set the world right.

With an exhale of relief, I hung up the phone. I had a headache. I could literally hear my heartbeat whooshing rhythmically in my ear, keeping time with the pain. I pressed a finger to my temple, took a seat on the couch, and watched as a cat hurried to join me.

Except for a purring cat, the tiny one-room home was quiet. And I looked around the space, the walls lined with dark wood planks, looking more like a cave than a home. But, be it small, it was peaceful. And when one comes from a past where screaming and negativity are part of the home décor, quiet is appreciated.

I felt blessed. Yet I had no tangible possessions. In fact, everything I owned, from my car to the couch, had been given to me by a caring friend or family member, all who wanted to support my fresh start. My mother had bought me the sneakers I had on; my sisters often left cat food bags on my door.

"We are loved, aren't we?" I reached down and stroked the cat asleep against my thigh. Tiny, white paws stretched out and kneaded my arm, eyes firmly closed.

I began to think about how many people in the world lack love. How many don't have a meal, a warm bed, a single person checking in to see if they're okay? And as I considered this, my heart swelled in both sadness and joy. I felt pain in the injustice of the day, how the dark side was clearly sabotaging a family 4 thousand miles away. How a well-laid plan to help many almost crumbled under pressure. And inside all that, I also felt joy. Because it's not over until we breathe our last breath.

Patricia and I are meant to share this story. The thought resonated, like an understanding that did not feel solely on my own. And as I sat there, the sentiment grew, suggesting we would have to fight for it. Darkness doesn't like the light. Negativity will try to stop us from sharing these words of love. But God always wins in the end.

CHAPTER EIGHTEEN

THE MOVE

"Life is more fun when two are involved."
~ **Journal entry, 2013**

"Will you join me on the drive?" I wasn't sure I heard her right.

When Patricia first shared her travel plans, she said a girlfriend would co-pilot the trip, said it would be like Thelma & Louise, only without random men and death. I was happy to hear that; I even joked about whether they knew how to change a flat tire. A lot can happen in 2,767 miles. Then she changed her mind said her stepfather would go with her, which was a better idea in my book.

"I thought you had someone already?" I hesitated, then quickly switched gears. "Yes, I'd be happy to help. The drive will be fun!"

THE MOVE

Fun? That's what I honestly thought. That a woman could leave her loved ones, move thousands of miles from her world, and somehow, we were going to have—fun!

How stupid could I have been?

And the beautiful scenery I anticipated began when my plane descended into Portland, Oregon's International Airport. "Ladies and gentlemen, if you're seated on the right side of the plane, you can enjoy the view of Mount Hood, or Wy'east as it's known, on our descent. Thank you for flying with us today, and we hope to see you on another JetBlue flight in the future."

As luck would have it, I was on the scenic side of that aircraft. And the pilot was right; Hood was awe-inspiring! It was only mid-October, yet the mountain was dusted with stark, white snow. I imagined the skiers were very thrilled.

Patricia had mentioned Hood before, usually whenever she told stories of home. Her love for the Greater Northwest pulled at my heartstrings, even more now that I could see its beauty firsthand and from the air. She had mentioned her love for skiing said that Timberline Ski Resort was her favorite place. She shared memories of friends and family antics on the slopes, afterward enjoying hot toddies at a chalet known as Timberline Lodge. And her eyes always sparkled when she told these stories, piquing my curiosity all the more.

The Giant in Me

"The lodge was built in the day of Franklin D. Roosevelt," she said, as we left the airport and drove across the bridge from Oregon to Washington state, "and more interestingly, the exterior terrain was the snowy backdrop to the movie *The Shining*."

Now that's cult-fiction at its finest! So I thought, suddenly plagued with visions of a frozen garden maze—apparently, not filmed at Timberline—and a crazed lunatic chasing Danny through the snow!

Danny? I wondered. *Coincidence?*

Because Patricia's home was a long drive from the airport, I felt compelled to fill the time. "Do you drive this every day?" I asked, admiring the twists and turns on a road flanked by lush woods and rushing rivers.

"Forty-five minutes, every day," she said with a grin, adding, "one way."

"Whew," I sputter. "And I thought my DC commute back in the day was bad!"

When we pulled into the little town of Yacolt, Washington, I felt transported back 50 years. A single road split the tiny town in half. At the first stop sign, I could see a town library, a single-level, red-bricked building on the right, and an overpriced gas station on the left. The town itself was encircled by a deep forest, and no matter which way you turned, the road appeared to drift off into the woods. This out-in-the-sticks surrounding made a city boy like me fidgety, and the soundtrack from *Deliverance* began to play in my head.

"What's in that direction?" I pointed straight ahead, which happened to be the way we were going.

"That's the Gifford Pinchot National Forest," she said as she took a left. "But we're not going that far."

And she was right, as a mere mile up the road, Patricia's three-story log cabin came into view. At first sight, my mouth dropped open. And as we coasted down a long, gravel driveway, I felt like I was admiring a piece of art; the closer we got, the more beautiful it became.

"Patricia, this is truly amazing."

Upon exiting the car, my eyes lifted upward, drawn to a group of Douglas fir trees circling the house like a protective front. They must have stood 100 feet tall, and I figured were just as old in years. And when my gaze shifted back to the house, towering at half the trees' height, with its green-tiled roof and A-frame front windows, my awe skyrocketed to yet another level.

What could have happened that made her want to leave this? I kept questioning as a sadness nudged at my soul.

"This must be so hard," was all I could say. And when she looked at me, her gaze misty, I felt compelled to ask, "Are you sure you want to leave all this?"

"Without love, it's just sticks." Her matter-of-fact tone snapped us back to the task at hand. And without prompting, we got right down to the business of moving.

First, I met the grey Labrador I had only seen on video.

"Brinkley, meet Dan," Patricia said, as she opened the front door and a dog raced forward to shower his owner with love. "For now, just let him come to you."

It turned out, other than a quick sniff, Brinkley ignored me altogether. And it took all my concentration to act like I did not care. Wherever we went—upstairs, downstairs, outside—Brinkley was always there, monitoring from the sidelines and, I felt sure, judging my every move.

As I stood there, trying not to make eye contact with the dog, and holding a trash bag open for easy access, Patricia asked whether I skied. I said, "No, thank you," as I could not visualize 300 pounds on stilts. And with a bent ankle bone ta-boot, I explained I'd just skip the skiing and head straight for the after-drinks, thank you very much!

"Someday, we'll go up to Mt. Hood and have a drink," she said while somberly looking around an increasingly empty home. Her eyes lingered over a piece of hung metal art, her expression void of emotion. And then, realizing I was watching, she flashed a quick smile.

"Well, for now, we'll enjoy the scenery on the drive. It will be amazing!" I tried to keep things positive as

THE MOVE

we packed the Ford Explorer, end to end and top to bottom, with boxes of belongings.

I carried bag after bag of shoes; I had never known a woman with so many shoes! And as I hauled another load—the edge of a heel penetrating through and digging at my thigh—I reminded myself I had begged for the honor to escort her from coast to coast.

I also reminded myself that Patricia was grieving. And my spirit felt heavy too, burdened from the pain I could see on her face. All the love in my heart could not fix this, not right now. I had truly wanted this drive to be a happy time, a way to move us closer. But I had been a fool. The timing was terrible, and she wasn't ready. So my heart would have to wait.

As we pulled on to I-84 headed East toward Boise, Idaho, I looked back at Brinkley, Patricia's Labrador. He was sitting like a little gentleman, his rear against a box and a shoulder to the side door.

"Would he like the window down?" I had not been around a dog since I was 8. And Turd's life was cut short when he ate a steak bone that he couldn't pass! Poor Turd, the name alone had to jinx him. And that's when I turned to cats.

Brinkley turned his yellow eyes my way, looking at me like I had no right to speak. Maybe Turd's ghost had warned him about his crappy name or my lack of doggie knowledge. I had no idea, but this dog knew I was talking about him; that was a fact.

The Giant in Me

"He'll be fine." Patricia casually answered, not bothering to look at the dog, whose eyes flashed from his owner to me, then back to his owner again.

Lord, I hope there's not a secret command for attack!

"I'm sure he's a good boy," I said, more for Brinkley than his owner, and I took notice of the way his ears perked in the rear-view mirror.

Smart dog! We need to be friends.

For a drive this long, the food had to be planned out. Because, though I weighed in at just under 300 pounds, I had my eyes set on 250. Fast road food would need to be limited, so at first, we packed a cooler full of healthy snack meats, like cooked chicken and steak. We even managed a few whole-grain sandwiches, for fillers, along with string cheese and low-fat crackers. Bottles of water cooled in a separate container, and I did my best to ignore my cravings for a Cola!

After 700 miles, we pulled over in Ogden, Utah, for the night, a unique town nestled against the base of the Wasatch Mountains. The mountainous range hovered over the city like a watchful parent. I could not tell whether the buildings were built low because of a city ordinance or the contrast to the mountains offered an allusion. But the town glowed under the streetlights, reflecting the idealist feel of a Thomas Kincade painting.

Patricia said nothing, and from what I could tell, she had seemingly missed the view. Because of the dog, we had a room in the back of the hotel. Patricia had booked one room with two queen beds, and while Brinkley led the way—as if the dog knew where he was going—I tried to work out the schematics.

"Where do I sleep?" I hoped to sound casual.

"There are two beds," she said as she stopped at our door and began to fumble with the keys. Brinkley looked up at me as if he had just realized the problem.

"And the dog?" I asked, and those yellow eyes that had been watching me earlier looked up to me, and I smiled, muttering a silent, *Please don't eat me.*

"He sleeps with me."

Thank you, Jesus!

As I sat on the end of the bed that I designated as mine, Patricia made house. First, she placed a bowl of food and water on the floor for Brinkley. And then, grabbing pajamas, she headed for the bathroom.

Are we having fun yet? So I thought as I watched the dog sniff his now-empty bowl, snorting with obvious disappointment.

While I had no problem sharing a room, my nerves were on edge. I had not been with a woman in a private setting for many years. And then there was the simple problem of evening schematics that bothered me, like that I usually slept naked. Obviously, that was out of the question. And though I was prepared, having brought shorts and a t-shirt, my body temperature runs hot, and in looking around, I found no AC unit!

The Giant in Me

This is going to be a long night.

30 minutes later, when Patricia exited the bathroom, I kept my eyes on the open journal book in my lap. A light smell of vanilla and bananas entered the room right behind her, a trail of feminine loveliness that I tried to ignore.

Correction, this is going to be impossible. I wrote the words to the page, dropped the pen in the binder, and clapped the journal shut.

"If you're done, I'd like to take a shower?" I may have been living like a monk, but I was well versed in the seemingly endless bathroom rituals of the average female. So it was always best to ask and not assume.

"Yup." She looked up from a book to add, "I'm good."

I'm glad you're good, I thought. *Because I'm a wreck!*

I took my time, enjoying a powerful shower head, a pleasant surprise for a low-budget hotel. When I stepped out, I focused on the other room. I heard neither rustling nor voices; only an eerie silence enveloped me.

As far back as I could remember, I'd had a six sense of the world around me. And at the age of six, on a sleepover at Grandma Nan's, I experienced the world's multidimensions firsthand, when something or someone took my hand in the night. I woke, startled but curious, and with the feeling of five fingers encircling my own. From my bed cot, I looked up to my grandmother and the peaceful rise and fall of Nan's chest as she slept. Then back to my hand, where the touch was now gone.

It was not a dream. How I knew this, I cannot explain.

For this was not a talent I've researched since, nor one that I've encouraged. I'm like that fictional boy in the movies, the one who sees dead people, and yet, he wishes he did not. Only it's not the dead I see. Instead, I feel a residue of a room not at peace—an uncomfortableness then churns my stomach and pricks the nerves. However, on this night, I got nothing as I gave myself over to the quiet, listening with all my senses. The room was at peace.

The unease must be me. I sniffed back a laugh.

And as I opened the door, a rush of cold alleviated the heat throughout my body. A glow from my bedside table lit the way, and I was surprised at the sight of Patricia, asleep and spooning Brinkley like a mother cradles a baby.

Have I been in the bathroom that long? As I pondered the time, Brinkley's eyes opened.

His gaze followed me, but he did not move. And I found myself impressed by his ability to understand the circumstance and the effort to not disturb his owner. So maybe it was true; dogs really are man's best friend?

God knows, had this been a cat—even my own loveable felines—the concern would not have been in my favor. My little girl cat would have been irritated that I was touching her, much less strangling her neck as Patricia was constricting Brinkley at that moment. And to do this touching without permission, well, that could warrant retaliation, say barf on my pillow later, or in my shoe. And I don't know why I did it, but I gave Brinkley a wave goodnight just before I turned out the light.

Three hours later, I woke up to Brinkley's nose a mere inch from my own!

My mind blinked, literally skipped, and my eyes desperately tried to focus. Before this moment, I had never realized that a dog's eyes don't glow in the dark like a cat's. And why this thought came to mind—stress maybe?—I cannot say. But when I scooted back to see Brinkley clearer, that darn dog did not move. Outside of an ear twitch, not one muscle flinched.

What the heck is this game, a challenge? I looked over to Patricia, who now slept with her back to me. "Shew," I whispered, flipping a hand close to his nose. He cocked his head as if a new angle might improve his understanding.

Our little interchange must have stirred Patricia because she called for the dog, snapping a finger over a shoulder. And on command, he jumped to the bed and settled with his back to his owner. He laid his head to his paws, eyes still focused on me. And I could have sworn I heard a cackle; for what better way to keep an eye on you, my friend?

THE MOVE

How could I sleep, with all this tension? And now, I had to pee. So I flung the covers off, stepped out on the opposite side of the bed, and huffed to the bathroom. For a moment, I considered whether I should sleep in the bathtub, but I noticed it was still wet. So, having finished my business, I headed back to the room. I took two steps and found Brinkley sprawled out in the middle of my bed!

Are you f$%&*%* kidding me?* The curse exploded in my head. And I'm not a man that uses colorful language much.

I considered my options, waking Patricia, again—not a good idea. The poor woman had been a wreck all day, tearfully texting her family the entire way from Oregon to Utah. I couldn't bring myself to interrupt the sleep she desperately needed. And in looking to Brinkley, professing his dominance in my bed, I did what all sensitive men in my position would do—I took a chair at the table.

For the rest of the night, I contemplated how to overcome Brinkley's apparent dislike. I couldn't place where the distrust began because he had all but ignored me while in their home earlier and watched as I helped Patricia pack and load the car. Throughout the drive, he took treats from me, wagging his tail like we were old buddies. Yet here I was, sleeping on a chair, while he laughed at me from the center of my assigned bed. I mean, he chose to leave the snuggles of his owner to come and taunt me! Lord knows, had Patricia been snuggling me, I would never go.

No, obviously, I have a problem. I contemplated, wagging a finger at Brinkley, who merely lifted his head. Then, as if accepting my challenge, he returned to rest his chin to his front paws. He wasn't worried a bit! He was in, and I was out; the rest was up to me. I had to make friends with this dog, who was more like a child to the woman I loved.

The question of how plagued me until sunset.

***

Two days later, after nighttime walks, treats, and mealtimes where I offered to feed the little beast (I say that with love), he began to warm up. At first, it was slow—a nudge here and there for a pat on the head, a rub against my leg while we walked. And it was about this same time when the mood of the trip changed, from solemn to excited anticipation.

"I can walk him," I cheerfully offered. "If you want to go inside and get us some food?"

By now, the well-planned meals were falling to the wayside. It was becoming difficult to find a grocery store and restock the coolers with healthy snacks. So we decided to fast food it from here on out, and somehow I just knew I'd regret it.

The Move

"Make sure he goes to the bathroom, please," Patricia said just before turning to head inside the truck stop.

I had noticed the green grass in the front of the building, and though I was not aware of Brinkley's preferences, this seemed acceptable. So, I walked him over to the plush area, and he quickly began to prance around.

Good, be quick, I thought, while noticing a family of four watching me from their position near the window. With cheeseburgers now spread out before them, the kids looked especially happy. The kids, two in all, were chowing down their meal. In fact, junior number one never took his eyes off us as he ate. I could feel him watching as Brinkley took his time in his choice of spot.

"Come on, buddy, surely you can go now," I huffed, glancing back to the family, and the now-laughing kids. Junior number one was leaning over on junior number two, pointing, his hysterics sparking the parents into action, pointing and mouthing words that I could not hear.

I felt embarrassed for them, and tried not to watch. Until the parental units turned their eyes on me, their gaze burning with a familiar glare of frustration, one I remembered well from my childhood.

"What in the world are they looking at?" I asked, turning back to Brinkley, who was now squatting for the biggest dump I'd ever seen a dog take.

The Giant in Me

I felt myself gag as it rolled out like a gallon of soft-serve ice cream onto the perfectly manicured grass.

"Oh no. No!" I prayed for it to stop. "Okay, you're done, let's go. Let's go, buddy."

I was slapping the side of my leg with one hand, while tugging on Brinkley's leash, trying to guide him out of view. Or at least away from families who were just trying to eat their dinner in peace, without dog feces. But the dog only took a few steps before he took position again.

"Oh, please don't," I begged him, but it was too late.

Brinkley clearly approved of the spot, and because he was committed to the finish, I could only shrug my apologies to the families forced to watch from inside the food court. A second later, the dog did a happy dance of sorts. He was scraping the grass with his back feet, while hopping on his front. It was a satisfied dance if I had ever seen one. In fact, it reminded me of the TV character on *Married with Children*. If Brinkley had high-rise trousers, he would have flopped down and shoved a paw under his belt in true Al Bundy fashion.

"How did it go?" Patricia asked, handing me a hot, greasy bag of food.

My stomach flipped. "Great. Everything is just great." I sighed, glancing over my shoulder to the shitter in the back. The dog's eyes were dilated, focused on the food in my hand.

Just what he needs, more ammunition!

The Move

We still had 12 hours before we were to arrive in Maryland. And now, far from The Greater Northwest, Patricia's mood lightened; her quirky sense of humor returned. We no longer drove in silence but instead talked about everything, from God to the future. I shared how I thought she'd make a great co-host on radio, and she should think about joining me on the air. I had been thinking about an all-Elvis radio program and had a tip on a new station where I might pitch the idea.

"Radio?" She openly laughed, which didn't spark hope, but I rarely give up.

"Wouldn't you want to do an Elvis program, spin nothing but our man's music?" I was counting on the familiar word "our," believing that Patricia would feel a personal connection to the man as most lifelong fans do.

"Maybe." That was all she said.

And as it turned out, it was just enough to spark my courage. Because the next thing I knew, words exploded from my mouth, sentiments that really had no place here, but I had been considering them for so long now, I could not retract them once they were given life.

"I love you, Patricia Lee. But you know that…."

The admission lingered between us, like a hung jury, contemplating but undecided.

I'm in for the long haul, I thought. *Go big or go bust.*

"I know, it's bad timing." I sighed, impulsively flopping a hand over the seat towards Brinkley, who flinched over the sudden act of affection. "But I figured we might as well clear the air before we get back on the road. I… I don't expect anything. I just want you to know."

Except for a panting dog, the cab was silent. Patricia smiled that particular grin, the one she pulled out whenever she's caught off guard—a distraction tactic, I felt sure.

"Thank you. And you're right, I've known for a while."

That's it? I waited. But she said nothing more. *I tell the woman I love her, and she tells me she knows?* I wasn't sure whether to laugh or cry.

"Okay, good. Good." I turned back to the steering wheel, and with a flick to the wrist, turned over the engine. The car roared to life. "You might want to know, your dog just took the biggest dump I'd ever seen in front of God and small children."

"And you bagged it up, right?" She retorted so quickly, I could only blink my answer.

Her laughter roared. And my head snapped her way, like a diva on a Vegas show stage who's just been cut out of the opening line-up.

"That's not funny."

She laughed harder. Tears streamed down her face, and my own humor rose to the surface.

"Okay, it's a little funny."

Chapter Nineteen

Second chances

*"You smiled, you laughed. Your spirit was felt.
You were full of love and kindness.
You made my heart melt."*
~ "Angel," a poem by Daniel Hawthorne 2014

THE FOLLOWING YEAR PASSED IN a blur. Outside of life's mundane responsibilities, I spent my free days showing Patricia the beauty of Maryland. We biked through the Antietam Battlefield in spring rain and lounged under a warm night's sky for movies under the stars. That summer, I made it a point to partake in Brinkley's activities, like swimming at Green Brier state park and many games of fetch with a favorite blue bouncy ball. In turn, Patricia loved my little feline family, especially my little girl cat, who curled around her feet on their very first visit.

"She's so cute! What's her name?"

I braced for the dreaded explanation. "Well, they were once homeless kittens," I began. "Originally, I wasn't going to keep them, just nurse them, but they needed a vet and the clinic wouldn't take them without names."

Patricia was smiling and stroking my girl cat, who now lay on her back, begging for a belly rub.

"So, quick-like, I blurted out the first three words that came to mind." I pointed to the little girl still soaking up Patricia's attention. "That's Wiener."

Patricia's expression fell flat.

"That's Beaner." I pointed to the long-haired boy cat, then to the most prominent male cat in the house. "And that's Teeny."

As was usual, whenever the cat-name topic came up, the explanation muted the room. The sound of purring contentment echoed as Patricia continued to focus her attention on my little cat. And at this moment, more than before, I wanted to disappear. Sitting across from me, Patricia now chuckled, and I thought about all the names I could have chosen—sweet pea, snow cone, marshmallow. Anything would have been better.

Why didn't I change their names?

"So, let me get this right." Patricia considered, ceasing Wiener's attention, who now pawed at her leg and begged for more. "You were asked to come up with three quick names, and those were the words that popped out of your mouth?"

I didn't even try to explain. I'd stopped doing that long ago, so I merely nodded.

"This little girl here is Wiener?" Then, suddenly and somewhat shockingly, laughter burst through the room. "*Weiner?*"

"I know," was all I could say as I watched Patricia return to rubbing little Wiener's belly, stroking her ears, and cooing as if it were a new introduction.

"Nice to meet you, Wiener!"

Please stop saying it. "I know it's bad."

As Patricia's amusement continued, she scooped my little girl up into her arms. "Don't you worry, little miss, we're going to find you a new name, I promise."

"I didn't even know she was a girl," I tried to no avail.

"Miss Wee. That will be your new name," Patricia finally said. "Wee, wee, mademoiselle."

And Miss Wee, as she was now crowned, showed her approval by snuggling further into Patricia's arms. Although I had to admit, little mademoiselle did suit her.

"And you, sir." Patricia's attention snapped to me. "You are forbidden to name any more pets!"

I smiled shamelessly. "Hey now, Turd was my favorite dog, and he loved me."

Life was magnificent, colorful, and alive! I had never experienced a closeness with another human being before Patricia, never laughed so deeply, relished in long talks or tearful admissions. And we did cry together, as we both had many regrets to share where our failed marriages were concerned.

But when Saturday night rolled around, we were seated happy and cozily against a slab of 50-foot mahogany, seconding as a bar top, at the 28 South pub. The place had swiftly become our spot for drinks and live music, and the staff knew us well, so we rarely had to order.

"Hello, love birds. One dirty martini and a Natty Bo draft coming up."

We both nodded to a delicate brunette, barely old enough to pour our drinks. But drawn to an aura of love and happiness, she radiated whenever she saw us.

"Sarah, please tell my girl that it's time to let the world know about *us*!" I coyly grinned, nodding to the young woman who had been our drink expert for the last six months.

Sarah smiled from the far end of the bar, where she drew a cold draft beer for another patron. She had long been on team Dan and TL, as I had nicknamed Patricia, but this game of tease was too fun, so I continued. "Just one post on Facebook, that's all I'm asking."

"You should see how he looks at you." Sarah leaned over the bar, her words low and just between us. "Put the boy out of his misery already and give him what he wants."

The Giant in Me

Now we're talking! I suppressed an urge to hoot and whistle. *So young and yet so wise.*

Patricia was blushing as she sat on the stool to my left, her shoulder pressing against my chest. And when she melted even closer, I knew I was going to get my way. And it was about time! Because, though our close friends and family knew about us, our mutual friends abroad, though suspicious, were still patiently waiting.

Everyone wanted the details. How did it happen? When did Patricia and I officially start dating? And yet even we couldn't say how it happened. When did we transition from work partners to lovers? The facts were lost in a cross-country move, a lengthy divorce, and so many of life's minor disasters that neither of us could pinpoint a timeline. In fact, we don't even have a memory of an official first date or an anniversary!

When people ask, "How long have you two been dating?" we both look to the other, each of us perplexed over the specifics of a story that cannot be the sum of one day or time.

Many moments led us to each other. And after years as that unhappy giant in the room, experiencing nothing, every moment shared in my new life felt intense.

By late 2014, Patricia had taken me to Dublin and then London, England, where we finally celebrated our love with those same friends I was once nervous about meeting in 2010. Life through Patricia's eyes was more vibrant than I'd imagined, if that was even possible. And because she had lived life like a travel blogger, courtesy of those well-earned travel benefits, I was introduced to the glamorous side of travel. Like first-class seats that lay flat on flights overseas. I was a newborn, amazed by champagne before takeoff and a dinner menu, complete with build-your-own sundaes.

It's true what they say—once you fly first class, you will never want to sit in coach again!

But it wasn't just the flying that thrilled me. It was strolling around the streets of Bath, England, arm in arm, in search of under-advertised bookstores. Coffee at quaint cafés, cobblestones under my feet, and tea for two at 4 o'clock!

We experienced everything together, and my thirst for travel grew as we lived out every day immersed in each moment. And by the spring of 2015, we both agreed there was still one place, near and dear to us both, that deserved—no, required—a do-over. Graceland.

The weather was damp when we landed in Memphis. As is typical in the south, the rain moved in and out so quickly, only small puddles were proof it had ever happened. While the sun was warm, the temperature was mild as we strolled around the grounds of Elvis's home. Though we had been here before, separately, the moment felt much more pronounced together.

We had come full circle, two lonely people finding happiness in a town they both admired. And while

I recited the horrors of pain and humiliation from my last visit, she shared happier memories of writing her second book, *Dream Angel*, across the street from Graceland. Memphis had been her escape from the stress of life and a marriage on the brink of destruction.

"Memphis makes me happy," she admitted, while snuggling closer, her arms entwined around mine as we walked.

Her happy place. The thought resonated. I understood that, up to this point, something had been missing in her relationships. And Memphis was where any Elvis fan can go to be happy, so it made sense that she fled here to find peace.

"Why didn't we meet in 2010?" Patricia asked as we admired a room lined with gold records inside the Graceland Plaza. "We knew all the same people and even went to the same events."

"I saw you," I pointed out, "but you didn't see me."

Letting go of my hand, she turned to face me. "What do you mean?"

I watched you talking. I watched you dance. My heart wanted to speak, but my mind said not a chance. Lines from a poem I'd written weeks ago came to mind. The emotions were fresh, memories of when I'd first laid eyes on my angel still resonated, but Patricia did not know the whole story.

"Remember the charity event, the night after the dance party, you donated funds to Cerebral Palsy?"

I waited until her eyes flashed with remembrance and then continued. "I was sitting right behind you and your family."

She covered her mouth with a hand.

I didn't feel worthy; I didn't feel right. So I hid behind my walls most of the night.

"I couldn't believe my luck. After seeing you the night before, and now I was one row behind you?" I reached out and reclaimed her hand. "So close, I could hear your conversation."

Her emotions swayed inside those green eyes I'd come to love, from wonder to remorse.

"How did I not see you?"

You smiled so pretty; you were shining bright. I will never forget that angel I saw on that cold night.

"I'm glad you didn't. That wasn't me."

"Yes, but…"

"No more regrets." I drew Patricia into my arms, holding her close and tight. "This is our time now. Let's make everywhere we go our happy place."

I felt her nod in agreement against my chest. And my heart swelled to a new level of contentment. One can only feel the kind of peace when you connect with a kindred soul, another person who sees the world as you do. When all of life's events resonate similarly, whether it's religion or a walk in the rain, it's profound and equally felt.

I never could have dreamed you would enter my life; you're the best gift I've ever been given. I thank God every night. These written words were my heart. And the poem tucked inside my jacket pocket evoked my need to share. *You make me so happy; you've given me love. You're my pretty girl always, my angel from above.*

"I have something for you." I gently pushed her back to look into her eyes.

Those green eyes that had always mystified flashed with a fleeting moment of apprehension. When Patricia's gaze averted, I only smiled. She could never hide for me. I understood her. I wanted to marry this woman, and yet she clearly wasn't ready.

"Don't worry," I chuckled. "This isn't a proposal. But it is my heart."

While she shyly grinned, I took out the papers. The poem had been written on two pages of legal-sized, yellow paper. It was folded and creased, and with coffee stains on the top right corner, it did not reflect an elegant gift. But it held my heart—private sentiments dating back to the first time I had seen Patricia to this very moment.

"I want you to know my feelings," I said, watching her closely as she opened the papers and began to read the first few lines. "And I'll wait for however long you need. But you're going to marry me one day, TL. I promise you that."

It took about five seconds before she registered "marry me," and her misty eyes shot up to mine, questioningly, like she wasn't sure she'd heard correctly and needed clarification.

"I'm not asking now." I laughed. "I'll know when."

"Your confidence, Mr. Hawthorne, is very sexy," she softly teased while slipping back into my arms.

While her emotions were hidden under my lapel, I felt her close to my heart. Patrons from all corners of the world passed us, curious eyes drawn to love, while Elvis's smooth baritone filled the room, serenading all.

"Well, I am irresistible, so..." I said, loud enough for the curious seekers to hear, and I felt a girlie slap on my back, followed by giggling from deep inside my jacket.

We took many photos on that trip, typical for a well-enjoyed vacation. There I was, standing sturdy and tall between the front pillars of Graceland. No one looked at me and thought to offer a wheelchair. No kind person offered to lend me a hand as I made my way to Elvis's graveside. While Patricia and I stood together, kind visitors took our photo, capturing these important and pain-free moments.

But there was still one photo from 2010 that haunted me; it captured a 650-pound giant sitting at a table in the guest lobby of Sun Studios. Because the recording company was famous for discovering such artists as Jerry Lee Lewis, Johnny Cash, and, yes, Elvis Presley, it was a necessary step, so I insisted on going.

The Giant in Me

The photo shows me sitting, solemn amongst the famous Sun Record crown logo, displayed on t-shirts and hats alike. And though this moment was important to me, only my frowning face will forever be cemented in time. So it was no surprise, when I asked Patricia to help recapture a moment and set the record straight, that she enthusiastically agreed.

"Okay, a little more to the right," I instructed, and Patricia shifted a small, wooden table, built for two. My gaze bounced from camera to the photo in my hand to the new moment in front of me. "That's it! That's it!"

At first, Patricia and I took selfies on our cellphone. But she knew what I really wanted, and soon got up to recapture the exact photo from 2010—me sitting alone, only this time with the biggest grin I could muster. I could feel my smile stretch my cheeks, a warmth radiating, not only from my face but my soul.

There have been moments on this journey, spanning from 2012 to 2014, when I felt incredibly proud of what I had overcome, for helping others hurting as well as myself. But at this moment, in Memphis, I truly felt like I had finally made it! Like all the wrong was now righted, and nobody could take that from me.

Even today, whenever I examine these conflicting pictures, the apparent divergence of misery and bliss before me, I feel my heart swell with gratefulness and dignity. To me, it's photographic proof of a life wasted, in opposition to being genuinely alive; living in full color was a choice.

The first photo reveals a deflated man in pain, not only in body but spirit. He looks like he's been lured there, is posing against his will, and now plots payback. While the second displays a man filled with contentment and thankfulness. This is the real Daniel Wayne Hawthorne, the man God created me to be, and I like him.

When people ask, "Are you really this happy?" I return to this photo and report, "The eyes don't lie."

Chapter Twenty

Conclusions

> *"I'm not a doctor. I have no plaques on my wall. I'm just a man on a journey to find health and happiness."*
> ~ **Dan Hawthorne, 2022**

"Daniel," Patricia called out. She had used my formal name, which meant what she wanted to talk business. "Who would you like to dedicate the book to?"

It was 2022, post-publication, and we had just wrapped up the final details, like the author's note and acknowledgments. It was all very exhilarating and new. For months, Patricia had been saying the last days would be stressful, with editing and proofreading well into the night, so I should keep busy while she managed the details. But, I admit, the book was always on my mind.

Conclusions

What will my mother think when she reads it? I wanted to make her proud. So much of my life was filled with the big dreams that I'd never quite mustered. I'd spent a lifetime telling Mom, "I'm going to do this, you wait and see." She'd heard so much talk and, I worried, not enough action. *Maybe she doesn't take me too seriously anymore.* I wanted to show her.

"The dedication should go to you, of course," I answered from the living room where I was busy distracting myself with an episode of *The Walking Dead*.

Patricia and I had recently moved into a new house, and the boxes taunted me from every corner, overflowing into the guest room. There hadn't been time to fully unpack, and I sure wasn't going to do it without the lady of the house. Of that, I was sure.

"Hello up there, did you hear me?" I paused, waiting for a response, but other than our fur kids, the house was silent.

If she disagrees, who will she have in mind? I pondered while I watched Brinkley tiptoe over the wood floors like he was on ice. "Okay, I guess I'm getting up," I said to no one in particular. The idea climbing our new staircase less than thrilled me.

However, I'd long ago learned that my beautiful co-author rarely asked questions she didn't believe she knew the answer to. So she was most likely gaging whether we were on the same page. But, just in case we weren't, I began to reconsider my words.

"You're awful quiet," I said as I rose from my chair, the same one crowned as mine the moment we decided to make this a cinema room. "Did you have someone else in mind?"

I could dedicate the book to Thomas The Boss Burge. As I took the stairs and headed to our office on the second floor, I considered the idea. *Thomas deserves this honor; he has taught me everything I know in a gym.*

Truthfully, there were many deserving people, from God to my family, Pastor Rick, and many close buddies, like Barney. The list was extensive. But the task was to dedicate a book, not my life. Which meant I wanted to name someone who had helped the book get into the hands of readers, and there was only one person.

Her back was to me when I entered the office. As usual, Patricia was lost in her work, fingers racing over a keyboard and ears mute to everything around her. I smirked at the sight of her, fresh and beautiful, but still in her pajamas. *The girl would write an entire book in her sleep clothes if allowed.* The thought humored me.

"I think the dedication should be to you," I said, and took humor over the sight of her shoulders bobbing, obviously startled over the sound of my voice. "But I want you to write it like this…"

The typing stopped. And when Patricia turned, her expression was one of curiosity, and my heart rate began to escalate.

Conclusions

And because I was two seconds away from losing my courage, I hurriedly blurted it out, "To Patricia, my angel, my soulmate, will you marry me?"

For years, I'd joked that she would marry me, and she would merely give a coy laugh—the giggle all men have heard when a lady knows a man's right but is unwilling to acknowledge it. They'd rather keep us on edge; it's more fun, like an innocent game of lover's cat and mouse.

And now, as a slow smile crossed her lips, I released a held breath, felt my body relax as every muscle lessened one degree more. And when I saw a spark inside those green eyes, I knew I was golden.

"That's perfect!" She clapped her hands. "It's a wonderful way to announce our engagement, and it's the happy ending we've wanted!"

Was that a yes? I deliberated as her attention flitted over my body, examining my hands, my pockets.

"I don't have a ring, silly!" I laughed. "The idea just came to me!"

When her eyebrows drew together, and her head tilted ever so slightly, I realized exactly what she was thinking.

"No, I mean, the idea to put it in the book just came to me. I'd wanted to propose for a long time."

You know this! I was sounding frantic now. And I hated that, so I was grateful when Patricia reeled me back from panic in outer space.

THE GIANT IN ME

"It's okay!" She jumped from her chair and came to me, drawing her body close, and if I'd had hair, the ends would have been tingling. "Besides, I hear radio Gods don't need rings when they propose."

***

Patricia said yes to matrimony. She said yes to so many of my dreams, such as radio. And she has joined me in co-hosting the all-Elvis radio program, the same one I fantasized about for years, *Blue Suede Connection*. We're now syndicated (at the time of publication) in 8 countries.

My instincts were correct; Patricia was a natural behind the microphone. And while I've shown her the thrill of broadcasting, she has shared the beauty of literature. A fair trade, even though *The Giant in Me* was a 10-year process, and I tease her that the radio show is only two hours.

"I wish we could have met thirty years ago," I often tell her. "We would have accomplished so much together." The truth is, we were meant to live our life, just as we did, surviving the pain, and using those lessons in our time together now.

But human beings question, don't they? We are pondering, searching souls, so it's normal to ask why when we're given a trial or suffer through the pain. We are flawed by nature. While I trudged through the valleys of life, I cried and complained. I tried to fight the seed of hate, to no avail.

CONCLUSIONS

From an early age, I had been taught to love—love our God, love others as well as ourselves. For once we lose the ability to love, hope goes too. And while in the throws of battle, hope for a better tomorrow may be all we have that keeps us going.

"Faith, hope, and love. But the greatest of these is love." 1 Corinthians 13 is the secret to a balanced and peaceful life.

As a 650-pound man, I'd lost all hope. And faith had died too. I cursed God, judged him, and even questioned his existence. And love? Well, only a hint remained, and I saved it for my family and pets. Just enough to keep me alive.

When I tell people Patricia's my angel, it's not because she saved me—God did that—but because she believed in me. Long before we were "us," she had the wisdom to listen to a small voice telling her to share my story.

"Stop what you're doing," she'd heard the whisper, "and take another path."

At the time, Patricia was happy with her current direction. She was in the middle of writing the third and final book in her angel series—a compilation of Eternal Flame & Dream Angel—and readers were waiting.

"I am not a writer of memoir," she had told me, but God knew better. She was the one for me, in more ways than either of us understood.

The Giant in Me

We chased away the sadness, healing together. I've seen her demons, and she knows mine. And that giant voice inside of me? Beelzebub has been silenced, and the darkness that had manifested out of hurt and rejection, well, it's gone too. I am love and kindness. I am full of compassion, created for good, not only by design but by choice.

And from time to time, I think about that giant. He was with me at the bottom. And, I have no doubt, if allowed, he'd be here at the top too. But whether I like him or not, he is part of me. Not genuinely evil but confused. If allowed, he'd lash out like a child, unable to fathom a world where acceptance is denied and judgement reigns.

I caged him. It's true. I did what was necessary, not as punishment but for my own peace. That dark voice in my head was the epitome of negativity, and I wanted solace. I'm often asked if I regret the years spent as a 650-pound giant, and I answer, "No, not at all." I would not be the man I am today, had I not suffered. The fight only fuels my compassion. And when I see another human being struggling, I see myself. I want to reach out and hug them, tell them they are loved.

We all have a purpose. We aren't here by chance. Your best days lie in front of you; reach for them with both hands. **It can be yours**.

Addendum

While I'm told my happiness is evident, I would be neglectful if I failed to mention that my struggle continues. I am a food addict. And I will always be a food addict.

However, it was during my time of new discovery that I thought I was cured. And like most addicts, I believed the battle to be won, and all I had to do now was get on with living.

False.

Sure, I still felt the itch to race through a drive-thru, but I controlled it. The cabinets in my home were not full of cookies and chips. I drank gallons of water a day, not soda. But as I suffered through the consequences that obesity had given me, like the pain in my lower back and my rolled ankles, my disgust grew. Small things began to bother me, like how I still wobbled when I walked, my gate shifting side to side like that of an obese man. How was it that I felt sorry for myself, after coming come so far?

I had just weighed in at 280 pounds! Wasn't that enough? What more did I want?

250. I wanted to be 250 pounds, and I obsessed over it. To the point of forgetting everything I'd been taught, like gratefulness and grace. And I began to focus on the physical instead of the spiritual.

ADDENDUM

"I hate my chin," I'd complain, slapping at the skin that once made up for second neck.

Was losing over 300 pounds really not enough? Was I now going to be unsettled if I didn't reach some magical number in my head? I knew these feelings were irrational, not to mention a blatant disrespect for all I'd gone through. But they were real, and they were attempting to gain a strong hold over my soul.

When Patricia and I traveled abroad, I began to make excuses to sit. Once again, I could not enjoy life to the fullest, and even passed on a castle tour in the Czech Republic, because it involved walking. And furthermore, the ankle pain had become intense, so soon, I found myself reverting to my old ways of watching life from a bench—and yes, eating.

The habit of comforting myself with food came back. Only this time, the destructive behavior was not lost to me. I understood what I was doing because I had lived the consequences before. So, when we got back to the States, I quickly booked ankle surgery—I was going to walk pain-free in no time.

Eight months later, and even after daily physical therapy, I was still wobbling. And worse yet? I had managed to gain back 100 pounds. After losing almost 400 pounds, can you imagine regaining 100 in less than a year? I wasn't even aware the body could gain weight so quickly!

THE GIANT IN ME

To this day, I am baffled by the mystery. Because while recovering from surgery, Patricia was my caregiver and took control over the food. We now shared a condo in Virginia, and though I was couch-bound, she cooked only good meals. There was no fast food. And obviously, I could not drive, so there was no way to sneak drive-thru, though I admit the idea of ordering online intrigued me. But I didn't even do that. And yet, I went from 280 to just under 380 pounds—in no time.

Here I am, I thought. *I am a voice of inspiration, and now look; my clothes are tight again. Even my ball cap doesn't fit. Did my head gain weight? Can that even happen?*

I felt a flash of disappointed, in my self. And again, my world was off kilter. Fearful of losing control, I turned to an old habit and began to journal. I hadn't written a word, not a feeling or sentiment, in over a year. But with nothing but time on my hands, I poured out my disappointment to page after page. And to test my emotional waters, I wrote the five things that I liked about myself, only to discover I was back to picking the obvious:

1. I am alive.
2. I am not alone.
3. I have a roof over my head.
4. My car started this morning.
5. The sun is out.

Addendum

How pathetic. The thought flashed before I could catch it, and I couldn't believe my ears; my internal voice of doom (Beelzebub) had not said a word in years! I almost didn't recognize him. As outside of traffic frustration, I rarely allowed negativity to seep in, and yet, there it was. As if the devil himself had popped out of the floor with a, "Here's Johnny!" and suddenly, I was back in the cage with him as cellmate.

With my heart racing, I flipped a page and tried again.

1. Patricia loves me.
2. The fur kids, including Brinkley, love me.
3. I am the voice of inspiration. People look to me for a daily dose every morning.
4. I don't care what the scale reads. I am not 650 pounds. I am not that man.
5. I am human. I falter. But I will not fail.

Better, I thought. Then I dropped my pen to the book, read over the words again, and felt a sense of relief wash over me. All was not lost; I was very much in there. I just needed to focus on what I knew worked.

For the next two weeks, I spent hours analyzing how this could have happened. I even journaled my daily food—not a routine I typically like, but it's one way to find the flaws. And by reimplementing all the food tips inside this book, I discovered that portion control remained the center of my problem. I had lacked a colorful plate, which should include lean protein, green vegetables, fruit, and low fats—and water! But I was failing on all points.

While my rule of thumb had been for every serving size to be no larger than a closed fist, I had been overfilling my plate. I was eating the right things, but my portion control was off balance. Instead of taking extra veggies or salad, when still hungry, I would load up on the starches, like rice and pasta. Number two: my water intake was down. For someone like me, who weighs over 200 pounds, my daily water goal was 100 ounces, and more, if I could manage it.

Once I combined all that information with my lack of exercise, it was clear how 100 pounds had come back so quickly. So now, it was time to fix it—again!

You may be asking, why am I divulging these failings?

Indeed, I did not have to, for I'm not proud of regaining 100 pounds. And I could have easily crossed this tidbit out and left you with the happy ending. But fluffy conclusions were not why I wrote this book. I have shared my story as honestly as possible, eager to help others realize that the process I've spelled out in this book can help. That I've done it now twice! That we (you and me) are the key to our success.

Cultivating positivity in our life matters.

Desiring the change and turning your own internal key is the first step!

Finding a way to get moving, even it's just walking around the block, is a start.

Cutting out refined sugars, adding water—in place of soda—along with portion control, makes the difference.

Healthy servings of fruits and vegetables are needed!

And lastly, by silencing our internal negative dialog, that giant voice of doom will disappear, and self-appreciation will change how we see ourselves and others. This was my path to a healthy life—and it worked!

No, it's not easy. But yes, you can!

And the most fantastic piece of this journey came when I realized how every aspect of my life began to follow the positive path I had forged. When I shut out the darkness, my spiritual life flourishes. I become closer to the God I worship, and I believe 100% that I was saved in order to give others love and support. We don't survive pain just for the Hell of it; we live it to help another who may one day struggle with those same demons.

But we cannot fight alone! We need each other's support and love to be successful. And by not understanding this simple fact from the start, I had merely cultivated my downfall, and fighting alone had only helped me to reach 650 pounds. At the time, I thought I was strong enough, and I failed.

Don't be me!

In a world where support systems are readily available, we need not struggle in solidarity. There are many groups on social media sites like Facebook and Instagram. Or, if that's not your style, try a hands-on club-like TOPS (taking off pounds sensibly). Their in-person meetings are in many US states and Canada, but their Zoom meetings can be joined from anywhere in the world! So again, we do not have to fight alone.

***

The lessons from backsliding were many; the most important came in understanding my food relationship. It still feels as if food is my friend. However, food and happiness do not go hand in hand. Simply put, I hold food in high regard; I enjoy talking about it, sharing it with others, and I look forward to any event where a great meal is being prepared. This has not changed. The difference comes in my understanding when this friendship is supportive and when it's abusive.

If I've had a bad day, a suggestion of a good meal can improve my mood. Is this abnormal? On a basic level, most people commune in this manner, opting to make a bad day better around the dinner table. Only for me, food was not just a gathering; it was love. And every day was an emotional struggle; therefore, food was not enough to patch the pain.

Even with the abundance of love I experience every day, food still gives me a rush of joy. But I have learned how to keep a healthy perspective. So while food is not a priority in my life, I don't punish myself when I enjoy it!

The mere fact that I accept I have a food reflex gives me control. I can walk away from a drive-thru on a bad day. I can drive past a milkshake-shack and go home to a chicken salad—and I do, even to this day. I can plan, what I like to call, a free day and control when I choose to have a favored meal—the meal does not control me.

And I realize it's impossible to explain what a relationship with food feels like to someone that experiences eating on a general level. Non-foodies, as I call those who eat only because it is time to eat, do not understand the mentality around obesity.

I understand that.

They ask, why not just stop eating? If it were that easy, the OECD (an organization for economic cooperation) would not have found the United States the number 1 obese country in the world. And we wouldn't have 36.2% of our population classified as obese.

It's obviously not that easy.

So, if you are reading this book, and you are not obese or a food addict—maybe someone you love is struggling, and the topic resonates—I applaud you! And if you take away one tidbit from these pages, I hope it's the understanding of a need for compassion.

Judgment fuels self-destruction.

And the world supports a fictitious version of life—the fake happy family, the fake success. Society feeds the ruse, like the model starving herself to a preconceived perfection of 36 by 26 by 36, to be pleasing to the world. Or the man, who stands under 6 feet tall, made to feel less than a man because successful men are tall, dark, and handsome.

So where does that leave the rest of us, the 90% of the world?

For many, eating becomes a coping skill for life. We never see the weight as it creeps on, often in years, not days. And when we do, the problem is deemed unfixable. So, we eat more. And this destructive behavior spans many addictions—alcohol, drugs, self-inflicted pain, the list goes on and on.

It's never too late! Never. N-E-V-E-R!

It may take a love-tap of awareness, which can come from the most unexpected of places. For example, "Dan, is there anything else in town to do other than eating?" I'd heard that plea more than once. Admittedly, it wasn't the most tactful way of pointing out the obvious, but it did get me questioning why my behavior was problematic; was I so different?

Listen, when a non-foodie ignores the food commercials during a favorite show, I am still listening! And it's in this fact that I understand why I am unique. And I'm okay with being different. I knew my fight

Addendum

would involve more than just controlling calories and exercise. I would need to explore my emotional state as well. And that was fine because, well, I simply wanted to succeed that badly! I had finally turned my key. But the battle is never over.

I've said it before, and it warrants repeating; the fight is for life!

Acknowledgments

It's difficult to describe what it feels like to be given a second chance at life, the gratefulness and wonder of sunrise now seen with new eyes. Where I once viewed life through messy blinders, I now appreciate the beauty of life. While the rain can awe, a snowfall stirs emotion, like a painter wielding a delicate stroke to a canvas. Nature calms me.

I have been blessed to have had such assistance on this journey. From teachers to supportive friends and family, I will try to list as many as possible in this place and hope I do not forget anyone!

First, a big thank you to my girl, my angel, and co-author, Patricia Garber. I call you my tita (that's Hawaiian for a strong woman) for a reason. You genuinely are courageous, and I could not have tackled this project without you! I'm so glad you hung in there, conquering obstacles and the doubt. Because you were meant to be my co-author, and obviously, God had much more planned for us when he brought us together.

Thank you for showing me the world through your eyes, for loving me, encouraging me, and believing that I could take on this challenge. They say that behind every great man is an even greater woman, and you are the girl-power behind all we do. I love you, babe.

Acknowledgments

To Thomas The Boss Burge, you are the man! I needed someone like you in my dark time. Someone with your enthusiasm for life, health, and wellness. Your drive to make your department thrive pushed and inspired me.

To Sarah, Mrs. Boss, thank you for sharing that big smile with me and everyone every day in that gym. For cheering me on and supporting Thomas, who, in turn, helped me. We both needed your spirit, and Thomas is truly blessed to have your energy emanating in his life every day.

I could not have asked for a more supportive team for ALL the staff and students at Hagerstown Community college! Your encouraging words and happy smiles made me want to succeed even more. I hope you know what a huge part you all played in my success. The battle was so much easier once I realized I was not alone. And because of you, I was not.

To Ann Carbaugh, if you had not reached out to Thomas and introduced him to an unfortunate man, I just don't know where I would be today. However, living happy may not have been the outcome. And for that, I will be eternally grateful.

And to the head of HCC, Mr. Bo Myers, I thank you for allowing Thomas to work with me, for trusting me enough to allow me to speak to your classes and inspire others.

To my family—my mother, Rose, my sister, Terri and brother-n-law Steve, my other sister Crystal, and my brother Bill and his wife Sue, I am sorry to have caused you so much stress and worry for so many years. I can only imagine how helpless you must have felt watching someone you love teetering on the verge of death for ten long years! I am sorry for all the times I said I would change and never did. For all the times I made you feel like your concern was a bother instead of a gift. Thank you all for never giving up on me!

Thank you to Sandra and Neal McWilliams for letting me join your (Patricia's) family. Sandra, I know I don't need to tell you this, but it warrants repeating, you have raised a beautiful, loving, and talented daughter. I know you are proud of her, and I understand why. Also, thank you for not turning me into the Italian Mafia the day I showed up in the Northwest to drive your daughter East! That was a tough day for all of you, and I stand amazed when I think back to how much you had to have believed in Patricia's better judgment to allow her to drive away with a stranger (me) that day. Patricia and I cannot wait for the day when you and Neal come our way to stay!

To my good friend Jim Whipp, known as Barney in the book, and the entire Whipp family. We are truly grateful for your friendship and support. You have been with me from the start, riding motorcycles down the streets of Hagerstown like a gang of "Lost Boys."

Acknowledgments

You are the Corey Feldman to my Corey Haim. And we have slain many dragons on the warpath to adulthood. And we will soon have another haunted Gettysburg Halloween adventure, building more memories to laugh and cringe over! Thanks, buddy.

And finally, thanks to all that have followed me since the start of my "Getting My Life Back" blog in 2012, to our Kickstarter program supporters. Your funding brought Patricia to Maryland many times over to begin the journey that brought us to what's inside these pages. No one could have guessed it would take this long for publication, but we hope you enjoyed the story you made happen. And we thank you!

The best part? It's not over yet! To further our effort in helping others set their own plans and goals for their journey, we will be releasing a sixty-day inspirational companion journal (The Giant Journal) soon. The announcement will be released via social media and emailed to our subscribers. If you'd like to subscribe to our newsletter/email list, please go to https://dan-hawthorne.blogspot.com to subscribe. In addition, enjoy future blogs and information concerning our soon-to-be-released "Getting My Life Back" podcast and radio show—a full hour of helpful tips by guests in the health and wellness world.

To you, the reader, I hope something in this book can help you along your own journey. If you are fighting, please don't give up! And if you see my name on a venue in a town near you, please come and let me help. We can share the positivity together.

The world needs more hope and inspiration. People need to know they're loved and make the changes they need to be happy. So let's discover them together!

I am forever grateful.

Dan Hawthorne.

PEACE

Follow Dan!
http://www.dan-hawthorne.blogspot.com
https://www.facebook.com/gettingmylifeback/
https://www.pinterest.co.uk/DanGMLB/_created/

To contact Dan Hawthorne:
gettingmylifeback@gmail.com

Book a lecture event at:
http://www.dan-hawthorne.blogspot.com

From Patricia Garber

When one begins a story, the ending often eludes the writer. At least that's my experience; the story tends to write itself, page after page, and the end comes in its own time. Each written paragraph is like a stepping-stone, leading to the final thought and the point as to why a reader has spent their days—and I hope, their nights—racing to the end.

When I started Dan's project, I knew the beginning—he had lived every minute of it—but the ending wasn't clear. As the years passed, Dan and I's relationship evolved and our life became one, so there was no clear end. *We* were really beginning.

From day one, Dan asked me to share our love story, along with his journey, inside these pages because he felt both were important. The idea that a lone woman in a foreign land can meet a lonely man and find happiness could give others hope.

I agreed with him. Our love story is unique. However, it was also years in the making with many hurdles to overcome. And what part of that was exciting, and what part was plain drama? That was the ultimate question.

You see, to me, the East Coast was really a foreign land. It's still inside the immense landscape that is the USA, of course, but to a woman who once lived amongst swift rivers and snow-capped mountains, big city lights did not impress me. And outside of Dan, it took years for me to see her charm.

When I first left The Greater Northwest in 2013, the stress from losing my marriage and my home, and my family's distance, emotionally crippled me. Depression, chronic illness, and writer's block were always present at my pity party.

I honestly did not think this book would ever finish, much less see publication.

Dan knew better. And through the months and years that followed of me not writing, he practiced patience and love. I had never seen a man such as this man, tender and optimistic to a fault. Whenever I cried, my cup was half empty; he would gently remind me that it was also half full and that life was only as good as you chose to see it.

I laugh when I think about this now, but this philosophy really ticked me off at the time. Not because Dan was wrong, per se, but because I wanted someone to get in the gutters with me and feel as hopeless as I did. I was not looking for cheer. I was busy walling in my beer, or wine, as that was more my drink of choice.

But he wouldn't wallow with me; instead, he kept telling me his story, a story of redemption and rescue. Remember, we were drafting a book together, so he managed to share these ideals without effort. Over and over, he kept insisting "energy goes where energy flows," reciting times when he had made it to tomorrow only because he was focused on light and not the darkness. How negativity was the devil's most significant partner, and the crime of the century was what he could steel right under one's nose — life, happiness, and peace, all of it and more were at risk.

Honestly, if it weren't for Daniel, I'm not sure how long I would have stayed in my own cave of sadness.

From 2014 to 2018, I worked on Patricia Garber. I was still not writing — it's often called situational writer's block, where a life circumstance stops a storyteller for a time. Even the great Stephen King admitted to four months of writer's block in his book *On Writing*, admitting to a period of not writing, drinking beer, and watching daytime soaps!

Okay, four months versus four years… When I do things, I go big!

Those four years were spent traveling and growing with Daniel, sharing my life and family with him, as well as co-hosting *Blue Suede Connection*, an all-Elvis radio show he swore I'd be good at. And I loved it, just as he said I would. Then 2019 came, and I woke up one day — yes, that's exactly how it happened — and I was ready to get to work.

So much of life was experienced in those years not writing; another story could be written on our travel experiences alone. But this book is not about that. It's about hope. It's about love. It's about understanding our value. And how, when we live in the light, we reach our full potential. It's about all that, and…it's about damn time!

Thank you for reading! And thank you, Danny-boy, for trusting me with your story. But mostly, I thank you for loving me through the worse time of my life.

Patricia Garber

~

OTHER BOOKS BY PATRICIA GARBER

Eternal Flame
(An Elvis Fan-Fiction Series) Book 1

She's been blinded by grief. He's the long-lost King of Rock 'n' Roll. Will their interlude on Earth end in a love for all time?

Samantha Bennett burns with anger. Bitter over her mother's death, the shy preacher's daughter has turned her back on God and is seeking escape on a girl's trip to Salem, Massachusetts. But after narrowly avoiding a terrible accident, the shaken young woman is moved by a fortuneteller's promise of a forthcoming handsome companion.

Stunned when Elvis Presley arrives as her guardian angel, Samantha embraces the adventure of the mischievous guide chasing some long-overdue fun. And as the strait-laced Southern belle helps the out-of-his time star navigate the complexities of modern life, she can feel her temperature rising when a spark of attraction starts to blaze.

Is a mortal falling for an icon utter madness, or is this a match made in Heaven?

Other Books by Patricia Garber

Eternal Flame is the first book in An Elvis Fan-Fiction Series of Christian romances. If you like sweet, good girls, charismatic heroes, and tales of redemption, then you'll adore Patricia Garber's blue-suede path to paradise.

Buy *Eternal Flame* to get all shook up today!

Also available in the series:
***Dream Angel* (An Elvis Fan- Fiction Series) Book 2**

Samantha's Secret (An Elvis Fan-Fiction Series) Book 3
Coming soon!

Available on Amazon.com!

Follow Patricia Garber!
- *https://www.amazon.com/Patricia-Garber/e/B006T3O61Q?ref_=dbs_p_ebk_r00_abau_000000*
- *https://www.wattpad.com/user/PatriciaGarber*
- *https://www.goodreads.com/author/show/891313.Patricia_Garber*
- *https://www.facebook.com/theangelicsaga*

To contact Patricia Garber:
- *eternflame@yahoo.com*

IN LOVING MEMORY

ROSE MARIE HAWTHORNE

*My heart weeps in your absence.
While also rejoicing, for I know you are with
our Lord.*
~ Daniel Hawthorne, 2022

JUST MONTHS PRIOR TO THIS book's release, my mother went to be with the Lord. She was ready to go, looked forward to seeing her daddy, my grandmother Nan, Aunt Thelma, and those dear souls I wrote about in this book. So much love had gone before her, and now soon to be reunited—she was truly thrilled.

Patricia and I had just moved into our new home, Virginia, and we'd been talking about Mom's first visit, the special meal we would prepare, while contemplating what Mom might say when she reads the dedication/marriage proposal at the start of the book.

Rose Hawthorne was a God-fearing woman, and when it came to her children, she longed for only two things in life; to hear we all loved the Lord, and that TL and I would soon be husband and wife.

TL and I spent hours going over the details, like where we would get married. "Some place easy for Mom," we both agreed. The talks were always about our moms.

And now, mine is gone.

Though she will not be in the physical, to enjoy all the good that is still to come in my life, her spirit will be with me. Of this I am certain. She was my biggest fan, my most vocal cheerleader. She wasn't the type that would grab you, draw you close, and tell you with her words. She was an action kind of woman.

I would hear of her support through friends. "I saw your mom, and all she talked about was what a great job you're doing, how you've really got your health back, helping others."

That was my mom; never one to tell me, but she would tell the world.

Those last days I spent with her, I talked while she listened. And I said all the things I knew she needed to hear, like I was good with God. And I choked back emotion when I told her TL and I were going to be married.

For a moment, she opened her eyes and a slight grin overpowered her. She loved my Trisha Lee, understood that God had sent her to me, and now she heard what she really wanted to hear—we were to be married.

When I explained to her how the rest of the world would find out, in a book dedication, she merely shook her head, not even surprised.

If I got anything from my mother, it was her sense of humor. For Rose Hawthorne loved to laugh. And my childhood is filled with memories of her sense of humor, like her tying cans to the back of my radio partner's car and writing "just married" on the windows.

"Dan, I think I just caught your mother vandalizing my car," he'd said, that deep voice breaking with laughter.

Alarm clocks under the beds at a women's bible camp, extra-large bars in my work lunch box, and brownies made with Exlax, offered to the neighborhood children responsible for papering our house with toilet paper — the antics went on and on.

I came by it honestly.

And she gave me her faith. Though, not always gently, as I was a strong-willed kid, who would find a way to ditch Sunday church, if allowed. The mother I knew lived for church. And the church we went to as a family was curious to me.

As I wrote in the book, the Evangelistic Temple filled this eight-year-old with vast amounts of humor. There was the speaking in tongues, which at first scared me to death. Until I learned to mimic the sounds, and then it was my favorite trick to whip out on the Church bus.

"Daniel Wayne!" Both Nan, my grandmother, and Mom would yell. But I could see them trying to hold back their laughter; they weren't fooling me.

"Are you going to wash old Mr. Peter's feet?" I'd fret, after observing the ritual, an act that was meant to humble one to another, but only appalled me.

"Now you know that women don't warsh men's feet." You never could take the Hagerstonian out of my mother, wash was warsh, and fish was feesh.

"Well, I hope you enjoy washing old Peter's feet," I'd continue, mostly because it made me laugh, never forgetting to add, "that's gross, Mom," incase she didn't know.

When at my largest, that 650-pound giant did not believe God existed. He questioned everything, argued the points of salvation over ever holiday, like, *If God really loved me, I wouldn't suffer as I do.* And, *If God is real, why doesn't he help me?*

My mother suffered through this time in my life, watching her son question everything she'd spent a lifetime instilling in all her children. And when given a second chance, by that same God, I told the world I was grateful. I shouted His praise, but I did not make it clear to Mom.

Honestly, I thought she knew. Through it all, it never dawned on me that she may have taken all my God-bashing seriously. I was just complaining like a spoiled child; I didn't really mean it.

And for as many conversations I'd had about God with TL, I wish I would have said more to my mother. Because on her death bed, this was what she cared about, whether her baby had found the Lord. And when I did explain, I couldn't shake the feeling that she couldn't hear me, or maybe she'd heard but she wasn't convinced.

Why do we wait to share such important sentiments?

"I guess I'm just private when it comes to God, Mom." I tried to explain why I had kept my feelings to myself all this time. "But believe me, God and I are buddies."

She passed away on a Saturday, the day before Valentine's day. Which according to my thinking, and all that is holy, meant her first day in heaven was on a Sunday. Now, how fitting is it that my mother should arrive on a day that no doubt includes a grand celebration in Heaven?

Not only was it her first day but it was God's day too, and I know she loved that day more than any other while here on earth. Well, that and Christmas; my mother lived for Christmas. But that's for another time and another book.

It was bitter cold but sunny on the day we laid her to rest. Her body now lies with all the great souls from my family—my father, who preceded her more than 20 years ago, her mother, my grandmother, Nan, who she missed dearly, my Aunt Thelma, and Pap too, who she talked about as we waited for the Lord to take her.

Their souls are all together now. And when I think about it, a peacefulness resonates. For I know my mother is exactly where she wants to be!

I'm going to miss you, Mom. Nothing will be the same without you. But, if God allows, I know you will check on us. And you will see your baby doing you proud, helping and giving to others, just as I told you I would.

Maybe you'll see, when I said, "The book is coming, the book is coming," that it finally came. And all was right in my tiny world. Then you can rest in the knowledge that we're all going to be okay.

I had the best childhood. All felt right in my world, and I was young enough to be unaware of anything different. I have you and Dad to thank for that. And I do thank you.

~ Journal entry, 2022.

Your son, Danny.

Made in the USA
Coppell, TX
22 October 2023